Phytochemicals

Aging and Health

Phytochemicals
Aging and Health

Edited by

Mark S. Meskin
Wayne R. Bidlack
R. Keith Randolph

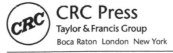

CRC Press
Taylor & Francis Group
Boca Raton London New York

CRC Press is an imprint of the
Taylor & Francis Group, an **informa** business

Cover art courtesy of R. Keith Randolph

CRC Press
Taylor & Francis Group
6000 Broken Sound Parkway NW, Suite 300
Boca Raton, FL 33487-2742

First issued in paperback 2019

ISBN-13: 978-1-4200-6137-6 (hbk)
ISBN-13: 978-0-367-38744-0 (pbk)

Library of Congress Cataloging-in-Publication Data

International Phytochemical Conference (6th : 2006 : Buena Park, Calif.)
  Phytochemicals : aging and health / editors, Mark S. Meskin, Wayne R. Bidlack and R. Keith Randolph.
    p. ; cm.
  "A CRC title."
  Includes bibliographical references and index.
  ISBN 978-1-4200-6137-6 (hardcover : alk. paper) 1. Phytochemicals--Physiological effect--Congresses. 2. Aging--Physiological aspects--Congresses. 3. Materia medica, Vegetable--Congresses. I. Meskin, Mark S. II. Bidlack, Wayne R. III. Randolph, R. Keith. IV. Title.
  [DNLM: 1. Aging--physiology--Congresses. 2. Phytotherapy--methods--Congresses. 3. Aged--Congresses. 4. Aging--drug effects--Congresses. 5. Plant Extracts--chemistry--Congresses. 6. Plant Extracts--therapeutic use--Congresses. WT 104 I603p 2008]

  QP801.P636I58 2006
  612.6'7--dc22   2008006053

Visit the Taylor & Francis Web site at
http://www.taylorandfrancis.com

and the CRC Press Web site at
http://www.crcpress.com

Contents

Michael Aviram, Mira Rosenblat, and Bianca Fuhrman

Sina Vakili, Grace Jooyoung Shin, and Marie A. Caudill

Marc Lemay, David Fast, Yumei Lin, Charen Buyce, and Lisa Rozga

R. Keith Randolph

Preface

Living healthier, longer lives is an almost universal value shared by most of the world's peoples. Both developed and developing societies around the globe are experiencing ever expanding populations of elderly and accumulating all the health-care burdens associated with aging populations. Interventions to help individuals remain healthy and active as they age are at the top of health providers' lists of priorities. Underpinning these public health and consumer interests is a large and growing body of research directed toward the science of healthy aging. A key component of this field of investigation is focused on elucidating the role of nutrition, plant-based diets, and phytochemicals in the aging process. This research has grown out of a substantial body of observational data pointing to lower risk of multiple chronic degenerative age-related diseases that are associated with the consumption of diets abundant in fruits, vegetables, and whole grains. Current research increasingly employs prospective and controlled clinical intervention studies to further elucidate the association between a plant-rich diet and a decreased risk of age-related degenerative conditions.

The 6th International Phytochemical Conference, "Phytochemicals: Aging and Health," was held in Buena Park, California on October 16 and 17, 2006. The conference was a joint effort of California State Polytechnic University (Cal Poly Pomona) and The Nutrilite Health Institute. This conference was the sixth collaboration between the two institutions, which have sponsored biennial international phytochemical conferences since 1996. Updated and expanded proceedings from the five previous international phytochemical conferences have been published: *Phytochemicals: A New Paradigm* (1998), *Phytochemicals as Bioactive Agents* (2000), *Phytochemicals in Nutrition and Health* (2002), *Phytochemicals: Mechanisms of Action* (2004), and *Phytochemicals: Nutrient–Gene Interactions* (2006). The organizers of the international phytochemical conference series invite well-known and respected researchers to discuss a chosen theme; "aging and health" was the theme of the 2006 conference. In each of the conferences, at least half of the presentations addressed the chosen theme. The remainder of the invited presentations covered new aspects of research methodology, real-world applications, and updates or expansions of previously introduced topics.

Presentations at the 6th International Phytochemical Conference began with a keynote address on prevailing theories of aging (Chapter 1), followed by discussions of state-of-the-art methodology with respect to polyphenolic analysis, bioavailability, and metabolism (Chapters 2 and 3). They continued with research presentations on botanicals and inflammation (Chapter 4), phytochemicals and vision (Chapter 5), phytochemicals and brain function (Chapter 6), green tea formulations and skin health (Chapter 7), and phytochemicals and cardiovascular disease (Chapter 8). The interest generated by the 5th International Phytochemical Conference, "Phytochemicals: Nutrient–Gene Interactions," led to a follow-up discussion on the potential for applying nutrient–gene interaction research findings to individual dietary recommendations (Chapter 9). The final two conference presentations provided discussions of commercialization of botanical products from concept through development and testing in the areas of allergy relief (Chapter 10) and inflammation (Chapter 11). The research presentations delivered at the 6th International Phytochemical Conference have been revised, updated, and, in some cases, expanded for this volume.

In Chapter 1, Timiras, author of the widely respected and extensively utilized *Physiological Basis of Aging and Geriatrics* (4th edition, 2007), gives her assessment of how we have achieved the recent significant gains in both longevity and quality of life as well as the problems associated with a rapidly expanding elderly population. In this chapter, Timiras challenges us to rethink our basic concepts of aging: "The now increasing evidence of the ability of older individuals to muster compensatory and even regenerative responses to aging-related changes well justifies a renewed theoretical and practical interest in the study of physiology of aging at the basic and applied levels." Timiras outlines six areas of research in the area of "life extension sciences" that have the potential to extend as well as to improve life in old age. One of the six areas is dietary manipulation, including a role for phytochemical medicinals or supplements.

Chen and Blumberg pose the following question in Chapter 2: "Are there age-related changes in flavonoid bioavailability?" These authors point out that a growing number of research studies have suggested that flavonoids may be linked to lower incidence of cardiovascular disease and some forms of cancer. They also make the important observation that "putative health benefits of flavonoids are critically dependent on their bioavailability, metabolism, distribution, disposition, and excretion—parameters that are now beginning to be fully characterized." While a great deal of discussion has taken place regarding the potential role of phytochemicals in disease prevention and health promotion, far too little discussion and research have addressed the pharmacokinetics of candidate phytochemicals. This failure to fully address pharmacokinetic issues has been a recurring theme in previous international phytochemical conferences and was addressed in several chapters in *Phytochemicals: Mechanisms of Action* (2004). Chen and Blumberg point out that "while the requirements for many nutrients change across the life cycle, data on the influence of age on the pharmacokinetics of flavonoids are sparse," such information is needed to understand the role of flavonoids in health and disease. These authors discuss what is known and unknown about flavonoid bioavailability and aging and suggest directions for future research.

As previously noted, epidemiological observations and *in vitro* studies suggest that not only polyphenols but also carotenoids may have health-promoting properties that might reduce risk of cardiovascular disease and certain cancers. However, as Koh and Mitchell point out in Chapter 3, "It is important to note that although flavonoids and carotenoids are implicated in the prevention of chronic disease, almost all attempts to assign health-promoting activity to the *in vitro* antioxidant action of any one specific compound of these phytochemicals have been unsuccessful." They also note that difficulties in interpreting intervention study data stem from such problems as "incomplete characterization of the test material, unvalidated biomarkers, and the lack of understanding of polyphenol bioavailability and metabolism." In order to move the science forward in this area, it is vital to understand and improve the analytical methodology for characterization and quantification of polyphenols and carotenoids. Koh and Mitchell discuss trends in the analysis of these phytochemicals and identify areas for improvements in this chapter.

The elderly segment of the population consumes the largest variety and the highest quantity of therapeutic agents. Dey and colleagues observe that "in the areas of cancer, infectious, and inflammatory diseases that are mechanistically linked, about 60–75% of the new drugs developed during 1983–1994 were based on naturally occurring compounds. This is in spite of the fact that a majority of the phytochemicals produced by the 250,000 plant species of the world still remains unexplored." These authors also note the disappointing track record of synthetic drug development over the same period of time. One explanation for the lack of phytochemical exploration has been the inability to apply high-throughput screening (HTS) techniques to multicomponent botanicals. The HTS methods have primarily been utilized to test single active ingredients. However, in a postgenomic era with so many potential targets and so much information available, these authors believe it is time to revisit screening and developmental approaches for botanicals. Chapter 4 provides "a case study for screening anti-inflammatory botanicals and strategies to further develop the identified hits into advanced therapeutic leads."

Chapters 5 through 8 discuss the roles of various phytochemicals in both healthy aging and chronic disease. Hammond and Renzi discuss the characteristics and function of lutein and zeazanthin within the human retina in Chapter 5. Age-related cataract (ARC) and age-related macular degeneration (AMD) are significant problems for the elderly. It is important to try to understand the role of macular pigment in the retina and its role in protecting the eye from diseases such as ARC and AMD. The ability of lutein and zeazanthin supplementation to increase macular pigment could impact retinal health. Hammond and Renzi provide a thorough overview of the current research and discuss the current hypotheses regarding protection from and prevention of disease in the eye.

One of the most common forms of dementia that affects the elderly population is Alzheimer's disease. In Chapter 6, Bastianetto and Quirion consider the possible neuroprotective effects of polyphenolic compounds. "Epidemiological studies have shown that consumption of fruits, vegetables, green tea, and red wine (in moderation) reduces the incidence of developing neurodegenerative diseases, including Alzheimer's disease. Polyphenols that are abundant in these foods and beverages likely contribute to their beneficial effects." These authors discuss hypothesized mechanisms for Alzheimer's disease and report on the results of experimental neuroprotective treatments utilizing polyphenols (particularly tea catechins and gallate esters).

In Chapter 7, Hsu discusses the possible preventative and therapeutic value of green tea in skin care and skin diseases. The author provides a brief history of green tea, identifies the key green tea polyphenols, reviews the hypothesized anticancer properties of green tea, and examines the prodifferentiation and anti-inflammatory properties of green tea polyphenols in skin cells. Hsu concludes that the experimental data "suggest that green tea polyphenols activate specific signal transduction pathways to regulate gene expression to accelerate terminal differentiation in the epidermis, in addition to their anticancer, antioxidant, and anti-inflammatory effects.

These effects not only are beneficial to many skin disorders, but also may provide anti-aging results."

Chapter 8 introduces a phytochemical source that had not been discussed at any of the five previous international phytochemical conferences. Pomegranate juice is a major source of polyphenolics and certain bioactive compounds in the juice have been shown to be bioavailable. Aviram and his colleagues provide a detailed discussion of the antioxidant activity of pomegranate juice polyphenols and review the results of studies of these polyphenols on the development of atherosclerotic lesions in both mice and humans. "All these antioxidative and anti-atherogenic effects of pomegranate polyphenols were clearly demonstrated *in vitro*, as well as *in vivo* in humans, and in the atherosclerotic apolipoprotein E-deficient mice. Dietary supplementation of pomegranate juice rich in polyphenols to patients with severe carotid artery stenosis or to atherosclerotic mice resulted in a significant inhibition in the development of the atherosclerotic lesions." Aviram and colleagues believe that their results suggest that combinations of antioxidants such as those found in pomegranate juice might be a better model for treatment than single antioxidants would be.

The 5th International Phytochemical Conference and the subsequent book, *Phytochemicals: Nutrient–Gene Interactions* (2006), generated a great deal of interest in nutrigenomics (the effects of bioactive dietary compounds on the expression of genes, proteins, and metabolites) and nutrigenetics (the effects of genetic variations on nutrient influences on health and disease of an individual). The field of nutrition science has always held out the hope of individualized dietary advice. However, for most of the history of nutrition science, dietary advice has been anything but "individualized." With the completion of the Human Genome Project and numerous research reports of nutrient–gene interactions, it may actually be possible to begin providing truly individualized nutrition advice. Chapter 9 explores this possibility; its objective is "to examine the feasibility, within the context of our current state of inquiry into nutrient–gene interactions, of using genetic information as cues upon which to base specific nutritional recommendations." The conclusions drawn by Vakili and colleagues are very interesting.

The final two chapters are an important part of the vision of the organizers of the international phytochemical conference series. The organizers hope to stimulate thoughtful and sound scientific research on the role of phytochemicals in disease prevention and health promotion. In addition, the organizers also want to encourage the development of commercial products based on solid research hypotheses and appropriate testing protocols. We would like to play a role in exposing industry to high-quality models of how to develop and test potentially valuable phytochemical products. Chapters 10 and 11 give two such examples.

In Chapter 10, Lemay and colleagues describe the development of a botanical combination product for allergy symptoms. First the authors describe a screening process to identify promising individual and combination botanicals with anti-allergic action. A selection of candidate compounds was then further screened utilizing skin-patch testing with human volunteers. The results of the second round of screening were used to formulate a potentially effective botanical combination formula. The finalized formulation was then tested in a double-blind, placebo-controlled clinical trial. Lemay and colleagues report on the outcome of this developmental process and suggest that it is "a model for achieving market entry and general market competitiveness of innovative technologies and products in the dietary supplement field."

Chapter 11 presents a different type of model for the development of an innovative therapeutic product. Randolph discusses the application of nutrigenetic principles (see discussion of these principles in Chapter 9) to the creation of a product that can modulate or positively alter certain physiological parameters in a person due to the existence of specific polymorphisms in that individual. One option (as discussed in Chapter 9) might be to make dietary changes, while another would be to develop a botanical therapeutic agent. In this chapter, Randolph discusses the development program strategy and the data from a pilot clinical trial.

We believe the research presented in this book should be of interest to a broad audience of food scientists and food technologists, researchers interested in phytochemicals, food industry innovators, nutrition scientists and nutritionists, and other allied health professionals. Phytochemical research is still in its infancy and it is the goal of these chapters to promote high-quality science and stimulate creative thought.

Mark S. Meskin

Acknowledgments

The editors and authors wish to thank The Nutrilite Health Institute, Access Business Group, for its support of the 2006 6th International Phytochemical Conference, "Phytochemicals: Aging and Health," held in partnership with the Department of Human Nutrition and Food Science, College of Agriculture, at the California State Polytechnic University, Pomona, October 16 and 17, 2006. The research presented at that conference contributed to the publication of this volume.

The editors would like to thank Randy Brehm for all her support and constant encouragement of this project. We would also like to thank Judith Simon and the editorial staff at Taylor & Francis Group for their patience and excellent work.

The Editors

Mark S. Meskin, Ph.D., R.D., is professor and director of the Didactic Program in Dietetics in the Department of Human Nutrition and Food Science, College of Agriculture, at California State Polytechnic University, Pomona. Dr. Meskin has been at Cal Poly Pomona since 1996.

Dr. Meskin received his bachelor of arts degree in psychology from the University of California, Los Angeles (1976), his master of science degree in food and nutritional sciences from California State University, Northridge (1983), and his Ph.D. degree in pharmacology and nutrition from the University of Southern California School of Medicine (1990). In addition, he was a postdoctoral fellow in cancer research at the Kenneth Norris, Jr., Cancer Hospital and Research Institute, Los Angeles (1990–1992). He received his academic appointment at the University of Southern California School of Medicine (1992) and served as assistant professor of cell and neurobiology and director of the nutrition education programs (1992–1996). While at the University of Southern California School of Medicine, he created, developed, directed, and taught in the master's degree program in nutrition science. Dr. Meskin has also served as a faculty member of the Department of Family Environmental Sciences at California State University, Northridge, and the Human Nutrition Program at the University of New Haven, Connecticut. He has been a registered dietitian since 1984 and is also a certified nutrition specialist (1995).

Dr. Meskin has been involved with both the local and national Institutes of Food Technologists (IFT) for more than 25 years. He is a past chair of the Southern California IFT and remains involved in the group. Dr. Meskin has been an active food science communicator for the national IFT, was a member of the IFT/National Academy of Sciences Liaison Committee, and has served as a member of the IFT Expert Panel on Food Safety and Nutrition. He is also involved in several IFT divisions, including the Nutrition, Toxicology & Safety Evaluation; Biotechnology; Nutraceutical and Functional Foods; and Religious & Ethnic Foods divisions.

Dr. Meskin served as a science advisor to the Food, Nutrition and Safety Committee of the North American branch of the International Life Sciences Institute for a 3-year term (2000–2002). He has been a long-time member of the advisory board of the Marilyn Magaram Center for Food Science, Nutrition and Dietetics at California State University, Northridge. Dr. Meskin was involved with the Southern California Food Industry Conference for many years as an organizer, chair, moderator, and speaker. He has also served as a member of the medical advisory board of the Celiac Disease Foundation.

Dr. Meskin is regularly invited to speak to a wide variety of groups and has written for several newsletters. He has been a consultant for food companies, pharmaceutical companies, HMOs, and legal firms. He is a member of many professional and scientific societies, including the American Dietetic Association (dietetic educators of practitioners; sports, cardiovascular, and wellness; women's health and reproductive nutrition; and vegetarian nutrition practice groups), the American Society for Nutrition, the American College of Nutrition, the American Council on Science and

Health, the Institute of Food Technologists, and the National Council for Reliable Health Information.

Dr. Meskin's major areas of research interest include: (1) hepatic drug metabolism and the effects of nutritional factors on drug metabolism and clearance; (2) nutrient–drug interactions; (3) the role of bioactive non-nutrients (phytochemicals, herbs, botanicals, and nutritional supplements) in disease prevention and health promotion; (4) fetal pharmacology and fetal, maternal, and pediatric nutrition; (5) nutrition education; and (6) the development of educational programs for improving science literacy and combating health fraud.

Dr. Meskin has coedited five books on phytochemical research, including *Phytochemicals: A New Paradigm* (1998), *Phytochemicals as Bioactive Agents* (2000), *Phytochemicals in Nutrition and Health* (2002), *Phytochemicals: Mechanisms of Action* (2004), and *Phytochemicals: Nutrient–Gene Interactions* (2006). He is a member of numerous honor societies, including Phi Beta Kappa, Pi Gamma Mu, Phi Kappa Phi, Omicron Nu, Omicron Delta Kappa, Phi Upsilon Omicron, Gamma Sigma Delta, and Sigma Xi. He was elected a fellow of the American College of Nutrition in 1993 and was certified as a charter fellow of the American Dietetic Association in 1995. He received the Teacher of the Year award in the College of Agriculture in 1999 from Cal Poly Pomona, the Advisor of the Year award in the College of Agriculture in 2002, and the advisor of the year award from Gamma Sigma Delta (national agriculture honor society) in 2004.

Wayne R. Bidlack, Ph.D., is a professor in the Department of Human Nutrition and Food Science and has return rights to the Department of Animal and Veterinary Sciences, California State Polytechnic University, Pomona.

Dr. Bidlack received his bachelor of science degree in dairy science and technology from the Pennsylvania State University (1966), his master of science degree in food science from Iowa State University (1968), and his Ph.D. degree in biochemistry from the University of California, Davis (1972). In addition, he was a postdoctoral fellow in pharmacology at the University of Southern California School of Medicine (1972–1974). He received his academic appointment at the University of Southern California (1974), serving as assistant dean of medical student affairs (1988–1991) and as professor and interim chair of pharmacology and nutrition (1991–1992). Dr. Bidlack has also served as chairman and professor of food science and human nutrition and as director of the Center for Designing Foods to Improve Nutrition at Iowa State University, Ames, from 1992 to 1995. He was appointed dean of the College of Agriculture at California State Polytechnic University, Pomona, serving from 1992–2007.

Dr. Bidlack has been a professional member of the Institute of Food Technologists for more than 30 years. He has served as a member of the annual program committee, as a member of both the Expert Panel on Nutrition and Food Safety and the Scientific Lectureship Committee, and as a scientific lecturer. He was program chairman and chairman of the IFT Toxicology and Safety Evaluation Division (1989–1990) and has served as a member of the Executive Committee for both the TaSE Division and the Nutrition Division. He has served as editor of the TaSE newsletter. For the Southern

California section of IFT, Dr. Bidlack has served as councilor, chairman of the scholarship committee, program chairman, and chairman of the section (1988–1989). He has also served as regional communicator for IFT in Southern California. Dr. Bidlack was elected a fellow of IFT in June 1998 and elected as counselor representative to the Executive Committee (2000–2003). He served on the finance committee (2003–2006) and as the chairman of the Strategic Planning Committee (2004–2007). Currently, he chairs the Audit Committee (2006–2009) and is chair of the committee on "making food safety decisions when the science is incomplete."

Dr. Bidlack is past president of the Food Safety Specialty Section of the Society of Toxicology, served on the International Life Sciences Institute Committee on Nutrition and Food Safety, and held the position of scientific advisor for the subcommittee on iron and health and the subcommittee on apoptosis related to fumonisin toxicity. He has also served as a member of the board for the Certification Board for Nutrition Specialists and actively contributed to the creation of the national certification exam. In addition, he is serving on the editorial board and as book editor for the *Journal of the American College of Nutrition*. He served as an editor of two books on phytochemicals published by Technomics and four others published by CRC Press; the seventh in the series is in press. He continues to review grants for several agencies and universities. Currently, Dr. Bidlack is serving as a member of the board of the California Department of Food and Agriculture.

In 1990, Dr. Bidlack received the meritorious service award from the California Dietetic Association and the distinguished achievement award from the Southern California Institute of Food Technologists. He was awarded honorary membership in the Golden Key, a national honor society, in 1995 and in Gamma Sigma Delta in 1998. He also received the Bautzer Faculty University Advancement Award for Cal Poly Pomona in 1998. In 2002, Dr. Bidlack was awarded the CSU WANG Family Excellence Award for Administrators. The Cal Poly Pomona chapter of Gamma Sigma Delta awarded Dr. Bidlack the outstanding faculty–administration award for 2003.

Dr. Bidlack's research interests are varied and integrate the general areas of nutrition, biochemistry, pharmacology, and toxicology. He maintains interest in the development of value-added food products, evaluation of biologically active food components (both plant and animal), and use of commodities for nonfood industrial uses. From these efforts, Dr. Bidlack has published more than 55 publications and 12 book chapters; he has edited seven books. He has been elected to several national scientific societies, including the American Institute of Nutrition (American Society of Nutritional Science), the American College of Nutrition (certified nutrition specialist), the Institute of Food Technologists, the American Society of Pharmacology and Experimental Therapeutics, and others.

Finally, Dr. Bidlack has served the food industry as a consultant in a number of areas, including as an advisor to the California Avocado Commission (serving on the Nutrition Committee) and the California Egg Commission on food safety issues.

R. Keith Randolph is the manager of the Analytical Services Department at Access Business Group in Ada, Michigan. He has oversight of a team of 44 chemists, engineers, and biologists who provide technical support for discovery, quality assurance, development, and manufacturing of consumer products distributed and sold through the Amway business worldwide. He has guided the planning and implementation of Nutrilite Health Institute's international phytochemical conference for the past 6 years.

Dr. Randolph came to Access Business Group in 2000 with 17 years of combined experience in teaching and basic research at the State College of New York, Stony Brook; the Medical College of Pennsylvania in Philadelphia; and the Cleveland Clinic Research Foundation in Cleveland, Ohio. He is first author on 18 original research publications in the areas of lipid biochemistry, metabolism, nutrient–gene interactions, cardiovascular disease, and skin physiology. He has served as editor for three books. He is a fellow of the American College of Nutrition. He also holds memberships in the American Society for Nutritional Sciences, American Chemical Society, American Society for Molecular Biology and Biochemistry, and the Association of Analytical Communities.

Dr. Randolph earned a bachelor of science degree in chemistry and biology from Wayland College in Texas. He also holds a Ph.D. in experimental pathology from the Bowman Gray School of Medicine at Wake Forest University in Winston-Salem, North Carolina. He was introduced to his scientific career in clinical laboratory science at the Armed Forces Academy of Health Sciences, San Antonio, Texas during a 4-year tour of duty in the U.S. Army between 1972 and 1976.

Dr. Randolph is the father of three sons, Matt, Parker, and Taylor, all of whom are in college in Texas. He is married to Susan Randolph, who, as a registered dietitian, shares his passion for nutrition and health. In his spare time, Dr. Randolph seriously pursues watercolor art. He extracts pigments for his art from plant materials, most notably flower blossoms. His art has been exhibited in New York and California.

Contributors

Anarbek Akimaliev
Biology and Soil Science Institute of the
  National Academy of Kyrgyzstan
Chuy St. Bishkek, Kyrgyz Republic

Jamin Akimaliev
Biology and Soil Science Institute of the
  National Academy of Kyrgyzstan
Chuy St. Bishkek, Kyrgyz Republic

Michael Aviram
The Lipid Research Laboratory
  Technion Faculty of Medicine
The Rappaport Family Institute for
  Research in the Medical Sciences and
  Rambam Medical Center
Haifa, Israel

Stéphane Bastianetto
Douglas Hospital Research Center
  Department of Psychiatry
McGill University
Montréal, Québec

Igor Belolipov
Tashkent State Agrarian University
Tashkent, Republic of Uzbekistan

Jeffrey B. Blumberg
Antioxidants Research Laboratory
Jean Mayer USDA Human Nutrition
  Research Center on Aging
Tufts University
Boston, Massachusetts

Charen Buyce
Access Business Group
Ada, Michigan

Marie A. Caudill
Division of Nutritional Sciences and
  Genomics
Cornell University
Ithaca, New York

C-Y. Oliver Chen
Antioxidants Research Laboratory
Jean Mayer USDA Human Nutrition
  Research Center on Aging
Tufts University
Boston, Massachusetts

Moul Dey
Biotech Center
Rutgers University
New Brunswick, New Jersey

David Fast
Access Business Group
Ada, Michigan

Bianca Fuhrman
The Lipid Research Laboratory
  Technion Faculty of Medicine
The Rappaport Family Institute for
  Research in the Medical Sciences and
  Rambam Medical Center
Haifa, Israel

Billy R. Hammond, Jr.
University of Georgia
Athens, Georgia

Stephen D. Hsu
School of Dentistry, School of Graduate
  Studies
Institute of Molecular Medicine and
  Genetics, Georgia Cancer Center
Medical College of Georgia
Augusta, Georgia

Eunmi Koh
Department of Food Science and
  Technology
University of California at Davis
Davis, California

Marc Lemay
Nutrilite Health Institute
Buena Park, California

Yumei Lin
Nutrilite Health Institute
Buena Park, California

Alyson E. Mitchell
Department of Food Science and
  Technology
University of California at Davis
Davis, California

Rémi Quirion
Douglas Hospital Research Centre
  Department of Psychiatry
McGill University
Montréal, Québec

R. Keith Randolph
Nutrilite Health Institute
Buena Park, California

Ilya Raskin
Biotech Center
Rutgers University
New Brunswick, New Jersey

Lisa M. Renzi
University of Georgia
Athens, Georgia

Mira Rosenblat
The Lipid Research Laboratory
  Technion Faculty of Medicine
The Rappaport Family Institute for
  Research in the Medical Sciences and
  Rambam Medical Center
Haifa, Israel

Lisa Rozga
Nutrilite Health Institute
Buena Park, California

Grace Jooyoung Shin
Department of Biological Sciences
Cal Poly Pomona University
Pomona, California

Ishimby Sodonbekov
Kyrgyz Botanical Garden of the
  National Academy of Kyrgyzstan
Akhunbabaev St. Bishkek
Kyrgyz Republic

Paola S. Timiras
Department of Molecular and Cell
  Biology
University of California, Berkeley
Berkeley, California

Sina Vakili
Department of Human Nutrition and
  Food Science
Cal Poly Pomona University
Pomona, California

Salohutdin Zakirov
Tashkent State Agrarian University
Tashkent, Republic of Uzbekistan

CHAPTER 1

Technophysiology, Evolution, and Aging
Toward a New Image of Aging

Paola S. Timiras

CONTENTS

TECHNOPHYSIOLOGY, EVOLUTION, AND AGING

The increase of human population and the extension of human longevity, both world-wide, represent perhaps the two greatest human achievements that have occurred from prehistoric to current times. In this introductory chapter, the biological consequences of this historical extension in human longevity are considered within the context of those factors and conditions that may contribute to promote longevity and quality of life in old age. Thanks to improving life conditions stemming from advances in agricultural practices, followed by progress in industry and technology, the life span has lengthened from 20–35 years in early history to 45–50 years in 1900 and to 80 years and longer at the beginning this twenty-first century.[1-3]

Thus, in the world's healthiest countries, approximately one-half of the increase in average life span has occurred during the twentieth century and persists in the twenty-first.[4] Continuing progress in longevity may be attributed to (1) public health reforms and improved hygiene, (2) advances in medical knowledge and practices,

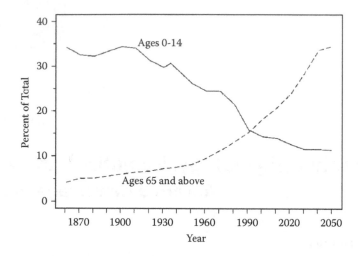

Figure 1.1 Proportion of the population aged 0–14 versus 65+ years of age, in Italy, 1861–2050. Note: The increase in the proportion of the old population has crossed over the decline in the proportion of the younger population in the early twenty-first century. Figures for 2001–2050 are projections. (From Timiras, P.S., *Physiological Basis of Aging and Geriatrics*, 4th ed., Informa Healthcare, New York, 2007. With permission.)

(3) better control of the environment, and (4) rising income and standards of living. Much of the increase in average life span has been ascribed not only to extended longevity, but also, in the most developed countries, to the near elimination of infant mortality (Figure 1.1).[5–7] Notwithstanding the improvement of survival at birth, the proportion of young people in the total population has decreased and continues to decline in most developed countries; this decline is primarily attributable to reduced fertility due to various socioeconomic and lifestyle factors. This is illustrated in the case of Italy, where the average family had five or six children in 1900, compared to one child currently (Figure 1.1). The challenge of a larger proportion of older than of younger people in the population demands "that societies reorient themselves toward the care of a large, dependent population at the end of life rather than at the beginning. Such adjustments are not without costs as the needs of children and of the elderly are quite different."[4] Therefore, careful social and biomedical adjustments and planning are required to provide for this significant shift in population distribution from younger to older ages.

In the United States, more people now live a longer average life span, and it has been forecast that this trend may continue.[5–7] For example, it has been predicted that by the year 2030 about one-fifth (18%) of the population will live to be 65 years or older (Figures 1.2 and 1.3). The increase—from 2.7% men and 3.8% women in 1900 to 15.2% men and 26.6% women in 2002—in probability that 50-year-old men and women may live to 90 years of age further illustrates the plausibility of this trend (Figure 1.4).

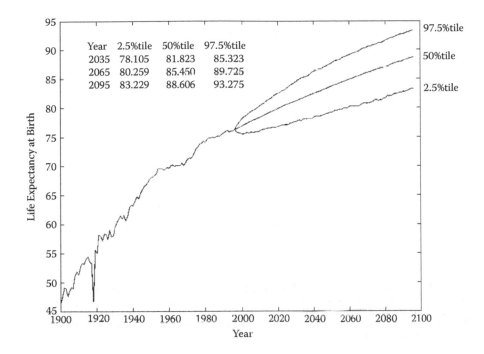

Year	2.5%tile	50%tile	97.5%tile
2035	78.105	81.823	85.323
2065	80.259	85.450	89.725
2095	83.229	88.606	93.275

Figure 1.2 Life expectancy at birth, United States, 1900–1996 (actual) and 1997–2096 (forecast). These projections are based on an extrapolative technique pioneered by Lee and Carter.[5] The inherent uncertainty of future trends is represented in the graph not only by plotting the median forecast (50 percentile) but also by showing two extreme forecasts (2.5 and 97.5 percentiles). (From Timiras, P.S., *Physiological Basis of Aging and Geriatrics*, 4th ed., Informa Healthcare, New York, 2007. With permission.)

To adjust to such a new and dramatic population shift, where the elderly represent an increasingly larger and even predominant group, is difficult but inevitable. Societies must rearrange their economic, technological, medical, and educational priorities. Such adjustments are as costly as they are complex because, while both younger and older persons are similarly vulnerable, their needs are quite different. Hence, if we are to achieve optimal social, economic, and medical support for both groups, any changes in priorities must be based on a solid understanding of the fundamental principles that regulate human aging.

With regard to old persons, in these early years of the twenty-first century, progress in medicine, hygiene, and biotechnology has led to a reinterpretation of aging as a positive process, free of the stigma it has had in the past of inevitable decline of health and productivity.[8–11] Until recently, attention had focused on the pathology of old age with the intent of combating diseases specific to this high-risk group. With the introduction of the concepts of successful and healthy aging, many researchers are shifting attention from a primary focus on the diseases of old age (the domain of pathology) to the possibility of strengthening normal function (the domain of

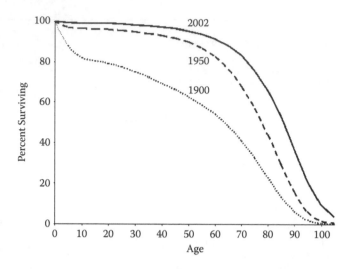

Figure 1.3 Survival curves for the U.S. population, 1990–2002. Note the lower survival in the age range of birth to 15 years in 1900 due to high infancy and childhood mortality in contrast to the progressive reduction of mortality in the same age range in 1950 and again in 2002. (Source: Arias, E., National Vital Statistics Reports, 53(6). Hyattsville, MD. National Center for Health Statistics, 2004.)

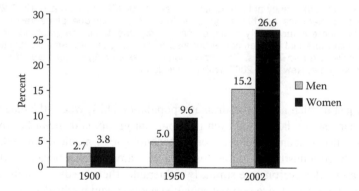

Figure 1.4 Probability of 50-year-olds living to 90 years of age, 1900–2002. Computed from U.S. life tables 2002. (Source: Arias, E., National Vital Statistics Reports, 53(6). Hyattsville, MD. National Center for Health Statistics, 2004.)

physiology and, more recently, of regenerative medicine) and prevention, in addition to treatment, of diseases.

One of the characteristics of the aging population is its heterogeneity, with some elderly individuals looking "younger" and others "older" for their equal chronological ages. This heterogeneity depends on both genetic and environmental factors

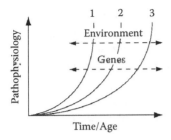

Figure 1.5 Schematic diagram showing that the life span is regulated by interactions between genes and the environment. The coordinates represent age from birth to death and the *degree of physiopathological changes* (generic for reduced function and increased illnesses) with progressively older ages. Three different curves illustrate the considerable heterogeneity in life trajectory among old individuals. (From Timiras, P.S., *Physiological Basis of Aging and Geriatrics*, 4th ed., Informa Healthcare, New York, 2007. With permission.)

(Figure 1.5). While representing a normal process, aging nevertheless would leave us increasingly vulnerable to a decline in physiological competence and an increase in risk of disease. In the United States, the majority of deaths from disease occur in the elderly, in whom diminished function makes the accumulation of pathological events less tolerable than in the young.

However, a growing number of current observations suggests that compensatory and regenerative capacity of cells and organs occurs not only in young but also in adult and old age in response to a variety of conditions (e.g., exercise, nutrition, learning). This is why the goal of maintaining or reestablishing optimal function, important at all ages, is particularly significant in elderly persons more susceptible to disease. Reciprocally, a strong function may prevent or delay the occurrence of disease and disability. Therefore, the second and third sections of this chapter will discuss compensatory and regenerative responses in the nervous system (a system until recently considered incapable of such responses) with respect to memory and neurogenesis, respectively. The last section of the chapter will present a brief list of present and future areas of research in the so-called "life-extension sciences."

THE THREE TRAJECTORIES OF LIFE

Early attempts to standardize functional profiles of old persons showed a progressive and irreversible decline in normal function. In humans, the physiological norm is exemplified by the sum of all functions in a 25-year-old man, free of any disease, with a weight of 70 kg (approx. 154 lb) and a height of 179 cm (approx. 5 ft, 8 in.). Comparison of old individuals with this "ideal" man inevitably discloses a range of functional decrements with advancing age (Figure 1.6). In trying to distinguish the elderly into discrete categories of varying degrees of physiological and pathological changes, it must be kept in mind that

1. there is great heterogeneity of responses among individuals of equal chronologic age;
2. changes do not involve all functions to the same degree and at the same time; and
3. the timetable of functional changes is differentially susceptible to specific intrinsic and extrinsic factors capable of promoting compensatory and/or regenerative measures.

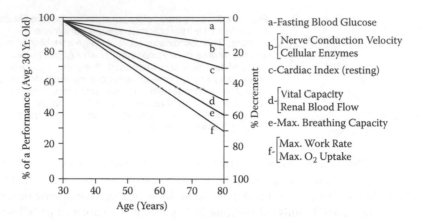

Figure 1.6 Decline in various functional capacities and physiological measurements of human males with progressive age (30–80 years). (Courtesy of Dr. N. W. Shock.)

Based on the substantive heterogeneity of the elderly population, a recent strategy groups the aging processes into three possible trajectories, thereby challenging the inevitability of functional impairment with aging[9,11]:

1. *aging,* with functional impairment, disease, and disability;
2. *usual aging,* with absence of overt pathology but presence of some declines in function; and
3. *healthy (or successful) aging,* with no pathology and little or no functional loss.

Examples of specific elderly groups that are undergoing successful or healthy aging have been selected and some of the lifestyles responsible for their success have been identified (Figure 1.7).

The concept of a single causative factor to account for some of the major life-span events pervades many areas of biological study, and gerontology is no exception. However, it seems unlikely, so far, that a single triggering event is responsible for the aging and death of the human organism; rather, aging and death probably entail numerous and complex biological interactions at different genetic and environmental levels. Functional competence for survival is indispensable at all ages. The now increasing evidence of the ability of older individuals to muster compensatory and even regenerative responses to aging-related changes well justifies a renewed theoretical and practical interest in the study of physiology of aging at the basic and applied levels.[11] In this chapter, examples of compensatory function are chosen from the central nervous system, a system hitherto considered incapable of any compensatory or regenerative plasticity except during development at a young age. Now, however, the nervous system is considered capable of undergoing plasticity and neurogenesis at all ages, as illustrated in the next section.

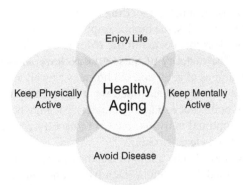

Figure 1.7 Health status and quality of life depend on multiple measures. Successful or healthy aging depends on a combination of lifestyles involving persistence of physical and mental functioning, avoidance of disease, and enjoyment of family and community support. (Courtesy of Dr. S. Oklund.)

EXAMPLES OF PHYSIOLOGICAL PLASTICITY: NEURAL COMPENSATORY AND REGENERATIVE MECHANISMS IN THE NERVOUS SYSTEM

Neural Proliferation in Selected Brain Areas

The adult human brain, a major component of the central nervous system (CNS), contains approximately 10^{12} neurons and 10–15 times that number of glial cells. On average, each neuron has 10,000 connections, resulting in an extraordinarily large total number of connections (about 10^{15}). It is through these connections that the CNS exerts its essential role of regulating communications between the organism and the environment and, within the organism, among the various tissues, organs, and systems.

Aging affects CNS structures differentially.[12,13] In the brain of old individuals without apparent functional or pathological deficits, neurons are not lost with advancing age or their loss is circumscribed to discrete areas:

1. The number of neurons remains essentially unchanged throughout life in the cerebellum and in some areas of the cerebral cortex, except perhaps at very old ages.
2. The number of neurons may decrease in some areas, such as substantia nigra (in Parkinson's disease), nucleus basalis of Meynert, the hippocampus, the adjacent temporal cortex, and olfactory pathways (in Alzheimer's disease).

Because of its involvement in the encoding of short-term memories and their conversion into long-term memories, the hippocampus has been the subject of numerous studies on the memory loss that occurs in the elderly, especially those affected with Alzheimer's disease. The majority of these studies have shown that new neurons develop in the hippocampus of adult and old humans as well as of experimental animals[14,15]; these studies have also determined what influences their genesis, survival, and integration in the brain. For example, neurogenesis may be stimulated by learning, physical activity, optimal nutrition, etc. to replace lost neurons or to facilitate recovery after brain trauma (e.g., stroke).[14–19]

With aging, there may also be a loss of dendrites and dendritic spines, a condition referred to as neuronal "denudation." Dendrites function as receptor membranes of the neurons and represent the sites of excitatory and inhibitory activity (further amplified by the spines on the dendrites). As the number of dendrites is reduced, synapses are lost, neurons are isolated, neurotransmission is altered, and interneuronal communication is severely impaired or no longer possible.[20] However, it has been demonstrated that new dendrites may grow or shortened dendrites may lengthen in different brain areas and lead to increased sprouting of synaptic contacts provided by the nearby neurons.[21] Such a compensation, perhaps less efficient than the proliferation of new neurons, persists in the old brain. One example can be found in the corpus striatum, one of the basal ganglia involved in the regulation of movement. The neurotransmitter of these striatal neurons is dopamine and the loss of dopaminergic neurons is considered the principal cause of Parkinson's disease. However, the alterations of motility characteristic of the disease become apparent only when half of the neurons have been lost; until then, reactive synaptogenesis of the remaining neurons is able to functionally compensate for their loss. Despite aging-related progressive striatal neuronal loss, disturbances of motility will become apparent only when reactive synaptogenesis is impaired or lost.

Several tissues renew continuously throughout life; this is the case with the bone marrow, the intestine, and the skin. It is now accepted that something very similar—neurogenesis—may occur also in the brain.[14] Neurogenesis starts fairly early in prenatal life with the transformation of actively proliferating precursor cells into new functioning neurons. The concept of adult neurogenesis has developed in recent years; it is based on the idea that development of an organ or tissue never ends and that adult plasticity, as manifested by neurogenesis in the adult brain, can be taken as the manifestation of continuing development.[22,23] Neurogenesis involves several events, among them the formation of new neurons and the securing of survival and supporting migration of neurons from the site of production to their final destination in specific brain function.[22,23]

Another type of compensatory mechanism available to the CNS at all ages is the proliferation of glial cells or "gliosis." Glial cells proliferate throughout life, including old age (Figure 1.8). Thus, both neuroglial cells (including astrocytes and oligodendrocytes), of the same embryological ectodermal origin as the neurons (see later discussion), and microglial cells, which are part of the immune system, proliferate rapidly in response to impaired function or damage or injury of the neurons.[24,25] The existence of neuronal precursor cells showing both neuroglial and neuronal

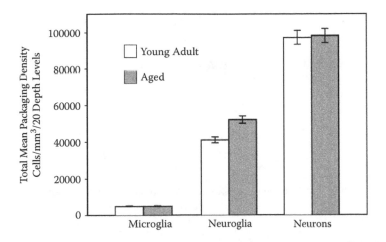

Figure 1.8 Mean values for packing density for total depth of cortex for a population of neurons and neuroglia cells (combined oligodendrocytes and astrocytes), as well as microglial cells in the cerebral cortex (primarily the sensory motor areas) of young (109–113 days) and old (763–972 days) male Long–Evans rats.[24] Number of cells of each type is indicated by the height of vertical bars, with the bracketed line (I) representing the standard deviation. Note the same number of neurons in young and old rats. However, the considerable accumulation of lipofuscin pigments in neurons, demonstrated by electron microscopic and immunofluorescent techniques,[25] suggests impaired metabolism. The increased number of neuroglia is then interpreted as a compensatory mechanism to support the function of the metabolically impaired neurons. Changes were not observed in microglial cells. (From Brizzee, K.R., Sherwood, N., and Timiras, P.S., *J. Gerontol.*, 23, 2389, 1968.)

characteristics has been demonstrated in several animal species.[26–30] Indeed, radial glial cells, which had long been considered to provide only a guidance structure for the migration of neurons, have now been identified, with astrocytes and oligodendrocytes, as part of the precursor cell pool itself.[31–33] Another event is differentiation into specific cells with a unique function. Therefore, interventions for promoting or inhibiting neurogenesis can be effective at different levels of development and aging.

Compensatory Mechanisms of Memory

Memory represents one of the functions regarded as the higher functions of the nervous system. Although these functions of the mind are numerous and range from motivation to judgment, cognition, language, and others, the focus here is on some aspects of memory acquisition, retention, and recall in young and old individuals.[34–36] A universal complaint among older individuals is the experience of not remembering as they once did. Impaired memory, often associated with aging, may range in severity from very moderate (as in benign forgetfulness) to major memory loss (as in dementia), as well as from transitory (as in delirium) to permanent and progressive (as in dementia of the Alzheimer type).[34–36]

Imaging techniques such as magnetic resonance imaging (MRI) are being utilized to measure increases in metabolic activity in response to the presentation of

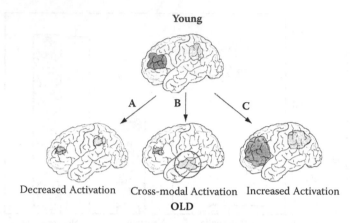

Young

Decreased Activation   Cross-modal Activation   Increased Activation
OLD

Figure 1.9 Different ways in which the brain activation detected by functional neuroimaging might vary between young (20–30 years) and old (60–79 years) individuals during performance of a cognitive task (e.g., remembering a number).[37] Although all groups performed the task well, the systems supporting performance differed between the two age groups. (A) A similar pattern of activation is seen in the two groups, but there is less activation in the old individuals in the corresponding brain regions (decreased activation); (B) a different pattern of activation is seen in the two groups, with new brain regions activated in old individuals (cross-modal activation); and (C) a similar pattern of activation as in (A) is again seen in both young and old but there is greater activation in older individuals. (From Timiras, P.S., *Physiological Basis of Aging and Geriatrics*, 4th ed., Informa Healthcare, New York, 2007. With permission.)

familiar visual clues.[37,38] Figure 1.9 presents a comparison of different ways in which brain activation may vary between healthy-young (ages 20–30) and healthy-old (ages 60–79) individuals during the performance of a memory task (remembering a number) as detected by functional neuroimaging.[37] Even though both groups performed the task well, the functioning of the neural systems supporting performance differed between the two age groups:

1. A similar pattern of activation is seen in both young and old groups in the same brain regions, but there is greater cell activation in the young individuals. This suggests that these same brain regions may not have been operating effectively as a network in older individuals. (A)
2. A different pattern of activation is seen in the two groups, with new brain regions activated in old individuals that are not active in young individuals. (B)
3. A similar pattern of activation is seen again in the two groups, but there is recruitment of a larger number of neurons to produce the same degree of activation in older individuals in the same brain regions. (C)

The recruitment of new brain regions in old individuals (findings 2 and 3) might represent compensation consequent to a reduced number of neural interactions or a lesser efficiency of the neuronal interaction; it is being considered as a compensatory recruitment of new neurons in the same or different brain regions, apparently in support of maintaining performance. Brain reorganization may be an inherent property of a normal brain that may be influenced by environmental factors and provide a way of compensating for changes that would otherwise cause a decline in cognitive ability.[15–19,38–40] This ability may be viewed as an expression of neural plasticity.

Neurogenesis from Neuroglia

As mentioned before, glial cells proliferate throughout life and actively participate in compensatory processes for repair, support, or, eventually, replacement of functionally impaired or lost neurons. For example, microglial cells are involved in a variety of actions pertaining to their function (e.g., anti-inflammatory) as immune cells. Neuroglial cells, comprising astrocytes and oligodendrocytes (Figure 1.10), derive from a common neural embryonic ectodermal cell that gives rise to both neuroblasts (and these, subsequently, to neurons) and spongioblasts (and these, subsequently, to astrocytes and oligodendrocytes).[41–46] Experiments *in vitro* show that addition to the medium of growth factors, such as fibroblast growth factor (FGF) or epidermal growth factor (EGF), stimulates neuroglial cell proliferation in a dose- and time-dependent manner.[47,48] Data from several laboratories suggest that these factors (as well as other growth factors) may "activate" the rapidly proliferating neuroglia to promote dedifferentiation of the adult cells into precursor cells eventually capable of differentiating into neuroblasts and neurons (Figure 1.11).

This process of transdifferentiation is preceded by a significant decline in the activity of those enzymes that are recognized as markers of neuroglial specificity. This is the case of the enzyme glutamine synthetase, the marker of astrocytes, which

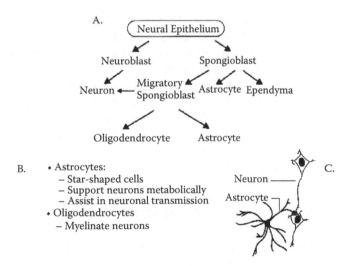

Figure 1.10 Some characteristics of neuroglial cells. A. The neural epithelium derives embryonally from the ectoderm and differentiates in neuroblasts and neurons and in spongioblasts that will differentiate in astrocytes, oligodendrocytes, and ependymal cells as well as migratory spongioblasts that may give rise to neurons. B. Major functions of neuroglial cells. C. Schematic shape of astrocytes and oligodendrocytes and their respective locations with respect to the neuron. (Courtesy of Dr. S. Oklund.)

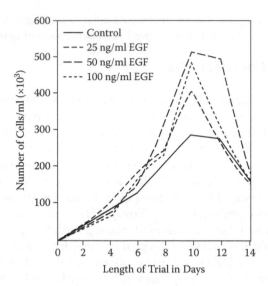

Figure 1.11　Growth curves of a mixture of astrocytes and oligodendrocytes from C-6 rat glioma 2B cells; the cells were incubated for 14 days with or without EGF (epidermal growth factor). EGF was added to the medium in three increasing doses. By 10 days, the cell cultured with EGF showed a statistically significant faster growth than the controls without EGF. By day 14, growth rates in all experimental cells had declined to control values.[47] (From Timiras, P.S. et al., *Mech. Ageing Dev.*, 126, 3, 2005. With permission.)

is reduced by 70% of the controls, and the enzyme 2′,3′-cyclic nucleotide 3′-phosphoydrolase, the marker of oligodendrocytes, which is decreased by 50%. Simultaneously with the decline in the identification of neuroglial markers, the cells express a progressive increase in the immunofluorescence of specific proteins Nestin and NeuN, which are well-known markers of neuroblasts (Figure 1.12). These markers were not present in the early neuroglial cultures but became manifest once they were reverted to precursor state and then to neuroblasts.[47,48] Studies in progress are investigating the electrical activities of these "activated" cells to determine whether they have, indeed, been transformed in functioning neuroblasts, endowed with the ability of generating vigorous action potentials upon stimulation.

FUTURE STRATEGIES IN BIOGERONTOLOGY

Maintaining or restoring a state of wellness in old age demands that physiological demands be strengthened and disease be eliminated. Although much has been accomplished in eliminating a number of diseases in recent years (primarily infectious diseases), much less has been achieved when it comes to basic function and preventing or repairing functional decline in old age. As discussed in several communications at the 6th International Phytochemical Conference in 2006, attention

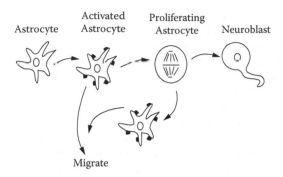

Figure 1.12 Schema of EGF stimulation of astrocyte proliferation and dedifferentiation into neuroblasts. Prolonged exposure to EGF causes astrocytes (taken as representative of neuroglial cells) to proliferate rapidly. It also causes them to lose their neuroglial characteristics, as shown by the decline in the activity of their specific marker enzymes; simultaneously, they will also reduce growth rate to control levels. They will eventually acquire precursor cell characteristics to become neuroblasts and neurons. Some of the proliferating astrocytic cells will maintain their characteristics, migrate to their usual location, and fulfill their usual functions.[47,48] (From Timiras, P.S. et al., *Mech. Ageing Dev.*, 126, 3, 2005. With permission.)

to a number of conditions in combination, such as appropriate diet, regular physical activity, judicious use of therapeutic drugs, and better education, are interventions that, in conjunction with strong economic conditions and social support, promote functional fitness at all ages.

The recognition that cells such as neurons and muscle or cardiac cells, which were previously considered incapable of proliferating in old age, retain the potential for plasticity and regeneration has opened the way to the study of intrinsic and extrinsic factors that may facilitate tissue repair in neurodegenerative diseases of old age. Likewise, the identification of pluripotent cells, such as stem cells, that are potentially capable of acquiring the structure and function of a variety of specialized cells promises to let us effectively replace lost tissues and functions.

Research in the area of "life extension sciences" purports to extend as well as to improve life in old age. Despite the controversial nature of some of these investigations, advances in several of the following areas continue to show a tangible and promising progress. They include, among many others:

1. The use of dietary manipulation:
   a. *Dietary caloric restriction* (CR) is a well-recognized way to prolong the life span and delay the occurrence of disease in a variety of experimental animals. In humans the possibility of "mimicking caloric restriction" by addition of supplements, fiber, micronutrients, and others that form the group of gerontoceuticals (i.e., potential antiaging cocktails that may mimic the metabolic or physiological effects of CR) bodes well for the possibility that the extended life and health spans associated with lower body temperature and insulin levels may ultimately be attainable without reduced food consumption or appetite.[10]

    b. Even in the presence of abundant food, the diet might not be optimal for ensuring normal function. Therefore, a *number of supplements,* including vitamins, minerals, polyphenols, and omega fats, might be very useful to provide essential nutrients. For example, recent studies from our and other laboratories show that curcumin, the biologically active ingredient from the Indian spice turmeric, has several well-recognized neuroprotective effects (e.g., antioxidant, anti-inflammatory)[49–51] as well as newly identified neurogenetic actions.[52]

2. Given the current "epidemics" of obesity, *prevention by education about optimal dietary regimens and eventual correction of abnormal eating behaviors, combined with physical exercise,* should be initiated at an early age and continued in old age.[53,54]

3. *A population of desired cell types that have the potential to produce new tissues should be generated.* The potential of embryonic totipotent stem cells could be exploited in the transplantation of retinal pigment epithelium, myocardial progenitor cells capable of restoring cardiac function and contractility, dopaminergic neurons for the treatment of Parkinson's disease, pancreatic cells for the treatment of diabetes, and others.[55]

4. *Cloning techniques to produce "human cloned body parts"* to be used as a source of young organs capable of being back-transplanted to replace failing organs in the older individual should be investigated. Nuclear transfer techniques proven successful for cloning goats, cattle, mice, and pigs may be applied to human clones, despite the potential risks of cloning and the strong ethical opposition.[56]

5. *Technologies to preserve tissues and organs for transplantation* and prevent tissue and organ rejection and for improvement of artificial organs and prostheses for replacing malfunctioning body parts should be identified.[57,58]

6. *New, improved, and genetically individualized pharmacological products for therapeutic purposes* should be developed.[59]

Another area of research that is progressing rapidly is the so-called *assistive technology.* This research utilizes a variety of engineering techniques to provide devices to monitor special functions of the body and provide detection and assistance if these fail—for example, the use of robots, the use of sensor "motes" (for recording of daily activity and eventual detection of falls), and improvements of *medical imaging technology* to further our understanding of function and diagnosis in treatment of diseases.[55]

While some of the predictions for life extensions may sound like science fiction, given the monumental changes that take place every day, these predictions are not that outrageous. Seeking immortality in the arduous old-fashioned way, doing good deeds, and taking care of one's children remain a goal worthy of pursuit, but need not halt efforts aimed at improving and lengthening life. Aging and death remain, indeed, the last sacred enemies—a fact particularly frustrating to humans who have now harnessed nuclear energy, circled the moon, decoded the human genome, artificially reproduced DNA, and significantly extended life expectancy. Such intrepid individuals can be expected to continue striving to improve the quality of life at all stages, as well as to extend the duration of life.

REFERENCES

1. Fogel, R.W. and Costa, D.L., A theory of technophysio evolution, with some implications for forecasting population, health care costs, and pension costs, *Demography,* 34, 49, 1997.
2. Fogel, R.W., Catching up with the economy, *Am. Econ. Rev.,* 89, 1, 1999.
3. Fogel, R.W., *The escape from hunger and premature death, 1700–2100,* Cambridge University Press, New York, 2004.
4. Wilmoth, J.R., Human longevity in historical perspective, in *Physiological basis of aging and geriatrics,* 4th ed., Timiras, P.S., ed., Informa Healthcare, New York, 2007, chap. 2.
5. Lee, R.D. and Carter, L.R., Modeling and forecasting U.S. mortality, *J. Am. Stat. Assoc.,* 87, 659, 1992.
6. Lee, R. and Tuljapurkar, S., Population forecasting for fiscal planning: Issues and innovations, in *Demographic change and fiscal policy,* 1st ed., Auerbach, A.J. and Lee, R.D., eds., Cambridge University Press, New York, 2001, chap. 2.
7. Lee, R.D., Rethinking the evolutionary theory of aging: Transfers, not births, shape senescence in social species, *Proc. Natl. Acad. Sci. USA,* 100, 9637, 2003.
8. Rowe, J.W. and Kahn, R.L., Human aging: Usual and successful, *Science,* 237, 143, 1987.
9. Rowe, J.W. and Kahn, R.L., *Successful aging,* Pantheon Books, New York, 1998.
10. Roth, G.S., *The truth about aging: Can we really live longer and healthier?* Windstorm Creative, Seattle, WA, 2005.
11. Timiras, P.S., *Physiological basis of aging and geriatrics,* 4th ed., Informa Healthcare, New York, 2007.
12. Filogamo, G. et al., *Brain plasticity: Development and aging, advances in experimental medicine and biology,* Vol. 429, Plenum Press, New York, 1997.
13. Freund, H., Sabel, B.A., and Witte, O.W., *Brain plasticity: Advances in neurology,* Vol. 73, Lippincott-Raven, Philadelphia, 1997.
14. Eriksson, P.S. et al., Neurogenesis in the adult human hippocampus, *Nat. Med.,* 4, 1313, 1998.
15. Fuchs, E. and Gould, E., In vivo neurogenesis in the adult brain: Regulation and functional implications, *Eur. J. Neurosci.,* 12, 2211, 2000.
16. Lowenstein, D.H. and Parent, J.M., Brain, heal thyself, *Science,* 283, 1126, 1999.
17. Berchtold, N.C. et al., Exercise primes a molecular memory for brain-derived neurotrophic factor protein induction in the rat hippocampus, *Neuroscience,* 133, 853, 2005.
18. Leuner, B., Gould, E., and Shors, T.J., Is there a link between adult neurogenesis and learning? *Hippocampus,* 16, 216, 2006.
19. Van Praag, H. et al., Exercise enhances learning and hippocampal neurogenesis in aged mice, *J. Neurosci.,* 25, 8680, 2005.
20. Scheibel, M.E. et al., Progressive dendritic changes in aging human cortex, *Exp. Neurol.,* 47, 392, 1975.
21. Cotman, C.W., Axon sprouting and regeneration, in *Basic neurochemistry,* Siegel, G.J. et al., eds., Lippincott-Raven, Philadelphia, 1999.
22. Kemperman, G., *Adult neurogenesis. Stem cells and neuronal development in the adult brain,* Oxford University Press, New York, 2006.

23. Taupin, P., *Adult neurogenesis and neural stem cells in mammals*, Nova Science Books, New York, 2006.
24. Brizzee, K.R., Sherwood, N., and Timiras, P.S., A comparison of cell populations at various depth levels in cerebral cortex of young adults and aged Long–Evans rats, *J. Gerontol.*, 23, 289, 1968.
25. Brizzee, K.R. et al., The amount and distribution of pigments in neurons and glia of the cerebral cortex. Autofluorescent and ultrastructural studies, *J. Gerontol.*, 23, 127, 1969.
26. Alvarez-Buylla, A., Theelen, M., and Nottebohm, F., Proliferation of "hot spots" in adult avian ventricular zone reveal radial cell division, *Neuron*, 5, 101, 1990.
27. Doetsch, F. et al., Subventricular zone astrocytes are neural stem cells in the adult mammalian brain, *Cell*, 97, 703, 1999
28. Kaplan, M.S., Environment complexity stimulates visual cortex neurogenesis: Death of a dogma and a research career, *Trends Neurosci.*, 24, 617, 2001.
29. Levison S.W. and Goldman, J.E., Both oligodendrocytes and astrocytes develop from progenitors in the subventricular zone of postnatal rat brain, *Neuron*, 10, 201, 1993.
30. Reynolds, B.A. and Weiss, S., Generation of neurons and astrocytes from isolated cells of the adult mammalian central nervous system, *Science*, 255, 1707, 1992.
31. Malatesta, P., Hartfuss, E., and Gotz, M., Isolation of radial glial cells by fluorescent-activated cell sorting reveals a neuronal lineage, *Development*, 127, 5253, 2000.
32. Noctor, M. et al., Neurons derived from radial glial cells establish radial units in neocortex, *Nature*, 409, 714, 2001.
33. Kriegstein, A.R. and Gotz, M., Radial glia diversity: A matter of cell fate, *Glia*, 43, 37, 2003.
34. Anderson, N.D. and Craik, F.I.M., Memory in the aging brain, in *The Oxford handbook of memory*, Tulving, E. and Craik, F.I.M., eds., The Oxford Press, New York, 2000.
35. Rosenzweig, M.R., Breedlove, S.M., and Levinson, A.L., *Biological psychology: An introduction to behavioral, cognitive and clinical neuroscience,* 3rd ed., Sinauer Associates, Sunderland, MA, 1999.
36. Agranoff, B.W., Cotman, C.W., and Uhler, M.D., Learning and memory, in *The Oxford handbook of memory,* Tulving, E. and Craik, F.I.M., eds., The Oxford Press, New York, 2000.
37. D'Esposito, M., Cognitive aging: New answers to old questions, *Curr. Biol.*, 9, R939, 1999.
38. Merabet, L.B. et al., What blindness can tell us about seeing again: Merging neuroplasticity and neuroprothesis, *Nat. Rev. Neurosci.*, 6, 71, 2005.
39. Adlard, P.A. et al., Voluntary exercise decreases amyloid load in a transgenic model of Alzheimer's disease, *J. Neurosci.*, 25, 4217, 2005.
40. Colcombe, S. and Kramer, A.F., Fitness effects on the cognitive function of older adults: A meta-analytic study, *Psychol. Sci.*, 14, 125, 2003.
41. Johansson, C.B. et al., Identification of a neural stem cell in the adult mammalian CNS, *Cell*, 96, 25, 1999.
42. Chen, S. et al., Dedifferentiation of lineage-committed cells by a small molecule, *J. Am. Chem. Soc.*, 126, 410, 2004.
43. Kim, S., Rosania, G.R., and Chang, Y.T., De-differentiation? What's next? *Mol. Interventions*, 4, 83, 2004.
44. Tsonis, P.A., Stem cells from differentiated cells, *Mol. Interventions*, 4, 81, 2004.
45. Itoh, T. et al., Cultured rat astrocytes give rise to neural stem cells, *Neurochem. Res.*, 31, 1381, 2006.

46. Seri B. et al., Astrocytes give rise to new neurons in the adult mammalian hippocampus, *J. Neurosci.*, 21, 7153, 2001.
47. Timiras, P.S. et al., The ageing phenome: Caloric restriction and hormones promote neural cell survival, growth, and de-differentiation, *Mech. Ageing Dev.*, 126, 3, 2005.
48. Thung, I. et al., Neuroendocrine regulation of proliferation, maturation, and de-differentiation of neuroglia, *Exp. Gerontol.*, 42, 146, 2007.
49. Cole, G.M., Teter, B., and Frautschy, S.A., Neuroprotective effects of curcumin, *Adv. Exp. Med. Biol.*, 595, 197, 2007.
50. Al-Omar, F.A. et al., Immediate and delayed treatments with curcumin prevent forebrain ischemia-induced neuronal damage and oxidative insult in rat hippocampus, *Neurochem. Res.*, 31, 611, 2006.
51. Xu, Y. et al., Curcumin reverses impaired hippocampal neurogenesis and increases serotonin receptor 1A mRNA and brain-derived neurotrophic factor expression in chronically stressed rats, *Brain Res.*, 1162, 9, 2007.
52. Panchal, H. et al., The antiproliferative and antioxidant curcumin influences gene expression of C6 rat glioma *in vitro*, *Exp. Gerontol.*, 42, 1, 2007.
53. Navazio, F.M. and Braun, M.M., Healthful aging: Nutrition and experimental strategies in dietary restriction, in *Physiological basis of aging and geriatrics*, 4th ed., Timiras P.S., ed., Informa Healthcare, New York, 2007, chap. 23.
54. Navazio, F.M. and Testa, M., Benefits of physical exercise, in *Physiological basis of aging and geriatrics*, 4th ed., Timiras, P.S., ed., Informa Healthcare, New York, 2007, chap. 24.
55. West, M.D., Bajcsy, R., and Timiras, P.S., Regenerative perspectives and assistive technologies, in *Physiological basis of aging and geriatrics*, 4th ed., Timiras, P.S., ed., Informa Healthcare, New York, 2007, chap. 25.
56. Lanza, R.P., Cibelli, J.B., and West, M.D., Human therapeutic cloning, *Nat. Medicine*, 5, 975, 1999.
57. Maathuis, M.J., Leuvenink, H.G., and Ploeg, R.J., Perspectives in organ preservation, *Transplantation*, 83, 1289, 2007.
58. Feng, S. et al., Transplantation in elderly patients, in *Principles and practice of geriatric surgery*, Rosenthal, R.A., Zenilman, M.E., and Katlic, M.R., eds., Springer–Verlag, New York, 2001, chap. 68.
59. Weinshilboum, R., Pharmacogenetics: The future is here! *Mol. Interventions*, 3, 118, 2003.

CHAPTER 2

Are There Age-Related Changes in Flavonoid Bioavailability?

C-Y. Oliver Chen and Jeffrey B. Blumberg

CONTENTS

INTRODUCTION

A strong, inverse association between the intake of plant foods, including not only fruit and vegetables but also nuts, red wine, green tea, and whole grains, and the incidence of chronic disease suggests they possess bioactive constituents with mechanisms of action that favorably impact pathogenic processes.[1-5] Indeed, the spectrum of phytochemicals, including alkaloids, carotenoids, phenolics, and organosulfur compounds,[6] possesses a diverse array of relevant bioactivity such as reducing inflammation, inhibiting oxidative stress, and modulating phase II enzymes. Flavonoids, a subfamily of polyphenols, are secondary metabolites involved in plant growth, reproduction, protection against pathogens and predators, and seed germination.[7] They are ubiquitous in plant foods and also components of many botanical medicines and dietary supplements. During the last two decades, flavonoids have been linked to a lower incidence of cardiovascular disease (CVD) and some forms of cancer in cohorts such as the Zutphen Elderly Study,[2,8] the Rotterdam Study,[9] and the Iowa Women's Study.[10] The putative health benefits of flavonoids are critically dependent on their bioavailability, metabolism, distribution, disposition, and excretion—parameters that are now beginning to be fully characterized. Interestingly, although the requirements for many nutrients change across the life cycle, data on the influence of age on the pharmacokinetics of flavonoids are sparse. This information is necessary to understand the role of flavonoids in health promotion and disease prevention. What is known about the relationship between flavonoid bioavailability and aging is presented here, with attention provided to important areas needing further research.

SOURCES AND INTAKES OF FLAVONOIDS

Flavonoids, products of the shikimate pathway from the phenylalanine and acetate pathways,[11] share a diphenylpropane (C6-C3-C6) structure of three phenolic rings (Figure 2.1). Flavonoids are ubiquitous in plant foods—for example, flavonols like

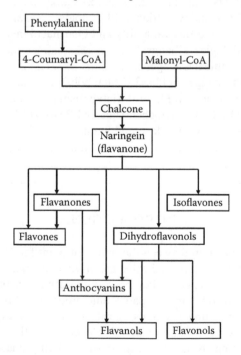

Figure 2.1 Simplified scheme of the flavonoid biosynthetic pathway.

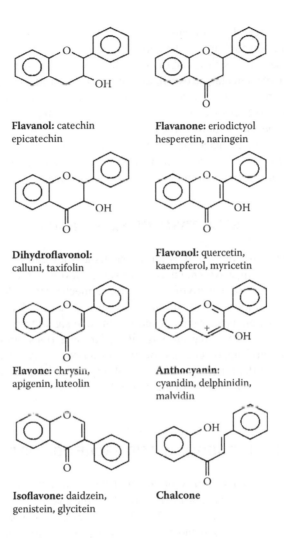

Figure 2.2 Flavonoid subclasses and names of prominent food flavonoids.

quercetin, kaempferol, and myricetin found in onions, kale, leeks, broccoli, blue-berries, red wine, and tea; flavones like apigenin and luteolin found in parsley, cel-ery, and cereals; flavanones like naringenin, hesperetin, and eriodictyol found in tomatoes, mint, grapefruit, oranges, and lemons; isoflavones like genistein, daidzein, and glycitein found in soy foods; flavan-3-ols like catechin and epicatechin found in green tea, red wine, and cocoa; and anthocyanins like cyanidin and malvidin found in red wine, grapes, beans, onions, and berries (Figure 2.2).[12] The majority of flavonoids have a conjugated moiety linked to the hydroxyl group via glycosylation, malonylation, methylation, and/or sulfation, with glucoside as the most frequently occurring conjugate in plant foods.[13]

Although an integral part of our daily diet, flavonoid intake has not been fully or precisely determined for nutrient databases because of the thousands of individual compounds present in this class and their marked variation in the same foods due to the impact of environmental, seasonal, and agricultural production as well as other factors like differences between varietals of the same species. Nevertheless, daily average intakes have been estimated to range from 96 to 600 mg/d, though individual differences may be substantially more or less.[14] Quercetin is among the most widely distributed flavonoids in plant foods; the average daily intake in typical Western diets provides 20–35 mg[15,16] and perhaps more as it is increasingly being employed as an ingredient in functional foods and dietary supplements.

BIOACTIVITY OF FLAVONOIDS

Flavonoids once were considered as antinutrients as they can bind and precipitate macronutrients and digestive enzymes.[13] However, flavonoids are now recognized as possessing an array of bioactivities with several mechanisms relevant to potential reductions in the pathogenesis of chronic diseases (e.g., anti-inflammatory and antioxidant actions as well as alteration of redox-sensitive signal transduction pathways and gene expression). While the investigation of these actions through *in vitro* and animal model research approaches has been informative, many of these studies have failed to appreciate the influence of bioavailability, metabolism, and disposition or of age—factors directly relevant to understanding the contribution of flavonoids to human health.

ABSORPTION, METABOLISM, AND EXCRETION OF FLAVONOIDS

Information on the bioavailability of selected flavonoid classes has been recently summarized.[15] Flavonoids are absorbed throughout the gastrointestinal (GI) tract and excreted in the feces or urine (Figure 2.3). The site and rate of absorption depend in part on the specific type of flavonoid and its conjugation, degree of polymerization, solubility, and food matrix, as well as the presence of other food components.[13,17] Conjugated sugar moieties are typically cleaved by lactase phlorizin hydrolase (LPH) or β-glucosidase prior to absorption.[13] Importantly, unabsorbed flavonoids may be degraded into phenolic acids by colonic microflora.[13] Once absorbed into enterocytes via active transportation or passive diffusion,[18] glucuronide, sulfate, and/or methyl groups are added to hydroxyl groups via the phase II detoxification pathway, principally in enterocytes, liver, and kidney.[12]

This biotransformation is common to many xenobiotics and diminishes the potential toxicity of the substrate and facilitates its biliary and urinary elimination by increasing its hydrophilicity. Flavonoid metabolites are transported to extrahepatic tissues and eventually to the kidneys, where they are excreted in the urine or incorporated into bile and excreted in feces.[13] Because phase II metabolism is highly efficient with respect to the flavonoids, aglycones (except for anthocyanins)

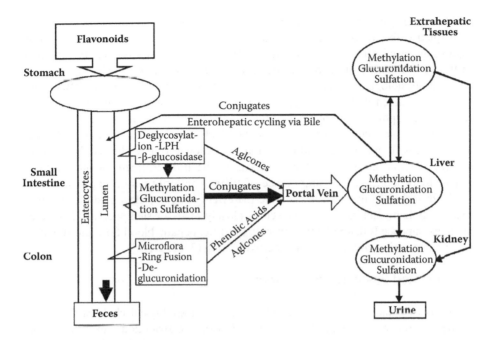

Figure 2.3 Absorption, metabolism, and excretion of flavonoids. Glucuronidation, methylation, and sulfation are catalyzed by UDP-glucuronyltransferase, catechol-O-methyltrasferase, and sulfotransferase, respectively. Abbreviation: LPH, lactase phlorizin hydrolase.

are generally absent or present in low concentrations in blood after consumption.[12] Many aglycones are produced via the action of β-glucuronidase in the small intestine, liver, and neutrophils[19,20] or by colonic microflora that can result in enterohepatic cycling of flavonoids.[12]

For most flavonoids, the maximum concentration in human plasma occurs 1–6 hours after ingestion with an elimination half-life ($t_{1/2}$) from 1 to 28 hours.[15,21] Therefore, flavonoids can accumulate in the circulation and in tissues with frequently repeated intakes. Plasma quercetin in free-living subjects, measured after overnight fast, is typically 50–80 nmol/L, though smaller values are observed following a low-flavonoid diet.[15] Conversely, supplementation with 500 mg/d rutin for 6 weeks increased plasma quercetin to 165 nmol/L[22] and to 0.63 and 1.5 μmol/L following supplementation with 80 mg and >1 g quercetin equivalents daily for 7 and 28 days, respectively.[23,24]

FACTORS AFFECTING FLAVONOID BIOAVAILABILITY AND PHARMACOKINETICS

The bioavailability and pharmacokinetics of flavonoids are dependent upon both the individual flavonoid and its food source as well as the individual subject.[13,17] In addition, macronutrients like protein and fats as well as other phytochemicals co-consumed with flavonoids can modulate their bioavailability, although information regarding these interactions is limited.[25–27] The significant interindividual variability in the bioavailability of flavonoids also implicates a variety of biochemical, physical, and physiological factors that may contribute substantially to these differences. Recently, Manach et al.[15] have suggested these interindividual differences may result from polymorphisms of intestinal enzymes, transporters, and/or phase II metabolism. Further, not yet well considered are the biochemical and physiological changes associated with aging and/or illnesses that are known to alter the requirement for several essential nutrients[28,29] but that have not been determined for flavonoids or other phytochemicals. The importance of filling this information gap is now recognized, including the need to examine the effect of age on flavonoid bioavailability, metabolism, and bioactivity as well as closely related issues such as age-related changes in phase II detoxification, protein binding, hepatic blood flow and function, body composition, and extrahepatic detoxification (Table 2.1).[30]

Age-Related Physiological Changes

Aging is associated with numerous physical and physiological changes that could influence flavonoid bioavailability, metabolism, distribution, excretion, and bioactivity. Compared to younger adults, the elderly have less lean body mass and water, serum albumin, cardiac output, gastric acid production, gastric emptying rate, gut motility, basal metabolic rate, liver size, hepatic blood flow, and renal function as well as more body fat (Table 2.1).[30–35] These factors, well known to variously affect both nutrient and drug actions, may similarly affect the putative health benefits of flavonoids across the life cycle. For example, changes in lean and fat mass dictate volume of distribution (V_d) in a manner inversely related to plasma concentration,[36–39] so the V_d of hydrophilic glucuronide and sulfate conjugates of flavonoids may decrease with age because of an increase in the fat/lean mass ratio. If plasma flavonoids are higher in senescent compared to young individuals, a faster clearance rate would be expected due to the positive association between $t_{1/2}$ and V_d. This relationship has been observed for aspirin, ethanol, lithium, and other drugs.[40]

Flavonoids can bind to plasma albumin,[41] possibly decreasing their diffusion into cells.[42] A 10% reduction of plasma albumin in older individuals[43,44] could impact flavonoid distribution to tissues; however, in fact, age-related decreases of albumin binding appear to have a minimal impact on the V_d of drugs.[45]

Aging is associated with marked changes in the structural and functional properties of the GI tract, including mucosal atrophy and reductions in pepsin secretion, lactase specific activity, villious area, splanchnic blood flow, and motility.[46–52] Woodhouse and Wynne[53] suggest that aging is responsible for moderate losses of small intestinal absorptive function, slowed GI transit time, and impaired mesenteric blood flow. Importantly, the age-related decline in LPH activity[52,54,55] may influence flavonoid absorption because of this enzyme's involvement in cleavage of sugar conjugates. However, with the sufficient reserve capacity of the GI tract,[37,42,48,56,57] these changes might have only a small impact on fractional absorption rates of flavonoids.

Table 2.1 Physiological and Biochemical Changes Relevant to the Pharmacokinetics of Nutrients in Older Adults

Parameter		Age-Related Changes
Absorption	↓	Activities of digestive enzymes
	↓	Bile flow
	↑	Gastric pH
	↓	Gastric emptying
	↓	Gastric secretion
	↓	Gastrointestinal motility
	↑	Gastrointestinal mucosal atrophy
	↑	Gastrointestinal transit time
	↓	Intestinal surface
	↓	Lactase-specific activity/lactase phlorizin hydrolase
	↓	Pancreatic trypsin
	↓	Splanchnic blood flow
Metabolism	↓	Basal metabolic rate
	↓	Enterohepatic cycling
	↓	Enzyme activity/inducibility
	↓	Hepatic blood flow
	↓	Hepatic mass
Disposition	↓	Cardiac output
	↓	Cerebral blood flow
	↑	Fat body mass
	↓	Lean body mass
	↓/↑	Membrane permeability
	↓	Serum albumin/flavonoid binding
	↓	Serum α-glycoprotein
	↓	Total body water
Excretion	↓	Glomerular filtration
	↓	Renal blood flow
	↓	Tubular secretion

Conversely, a prolonged GI transit could increase time for flavonoid absorption and metabolism. However, no studies have yet examined these relationships.

Age-related changes in the liver, including decrements of 30% in mass, 35–55% in blood flow, and 12% in bile flow, can affect the capacity for phase II metabolism.[52,58,59] These reductions impact drug metabolism[60,61] but a similar impact on flavonoid metabolism has not been explored. While the influence of these changes is less significant for drugs with a low extraction fraction,[62] the characteristics of flavonoids in this regard have not been established. Nonetheless, changes in detoxification enzyme capacity in the liver or other tissues could contribute significantly to an alteration of flavonoid metabolism and excretion with age.

Age-Related Biochemical Changes

In vivo and *in vitro* studies reveal that aging influences the bioactivity and toxicity of xenobiotics in part by affecting their biotransformation.[62,63] Thus, age-related changes in these enzymes may also impact the metabolism of flavonoids and, in turn, their bioactivity. Both phase I and II metabolism serve to increase water solubility and excretion of their substrates.[64] Phase I reactions typically involve oxidation, reduction, hydrolysis, and demethylation, principally via the cytochrome P450 system. Phase II pathways involve conjugation reactions in the cytoplasm, lysosomes, and endoplasmic reticulum with polar acetyl, glutathione, glucuronide, glycine, methyl, and sulfate moieties, with glucuronidation being the most common of these reactions.[30,37] Flavonoids appear to be metabolized primarily via phase II pathways. Interestingly, age-related decreases in xenobiotic metabolism appear to account for >80% of the toxic reactions to drugs in elderly patients.[52]

Age-Related Changes in Phase II Metabolism

Phase II enzymes involve the UDP-glucuronyltransferase (UGT) superfamily, cytosolic sulfotransferases (SULT), and catechol-O-methyltransferase (COMT) to add conjugates to functionally reactive polar groups, such as the hydroxyl moieties in flavonoids. Microsomal UGT are classified as the UGT1 and UGT2 families and metabolize >350 individual compounds with UDP-glucuronic acid as the donor.[65,66] UGT1 enzymes principally glucuronidate xenobiotics, while UGT2 enzymes catalyze endogenous compounds like steroid hormones and bile acids. However, the UGT1A1 metabolizes bilirubin, catechol estrogens, and flavonoids.[67] Glucuronidation capacity is prominent in the liver, but UGT activity toward bile acids, bilirubin, and phenols is also present in the GI tract and kidney.[66] Like UGT, cytosolic SULT comprises isoforms, with SULT1A1 (P-PST) involved in the sulfation of most phenolics, due to its broad substrate tolerance and high level of expression.[64,68] SULT catalyzes the transfer of sulfate, donated by 3'-phophoadenosine-5'-phosphosulfate, to hydroxyl groups of flavonoids. Differential expression is apparent in SULT isoforms; for example, SULT1A3 (M-PST) is expressed mainly in the intestine.[64,69] The cytosolic COMT catalyzes a wide variety of catechols, including catecholamines and estrogens, using S-adenosyl-L-methionine as a methyl donor.[70] The highest content of COMT is in the liver with substantial levels also found in the kidney and GI tract.[70] COMT biotransformation of flavonoids appears to occur at a higher rate than that of endogenous catechols.[30]

It is not clear whether the capacity for glucuronidation is preserved with age.[30,61] For example, Herd et al.[71] showed age did not alter *in vitro* glucuronidation or sulfation of acetaminophen in microsomal and cytosolic fractions of human liver cells collected from 22 subjects aged 40 to 89 years, although the lack of statistical significance in this study could be attributed to its small sample size. In contrast, Hansen and Stentoft[72] reported an age-related decrease in UGT activity toward dopamine antagonists, odapipam and berupipam in 17 human subjects. Using rodent models, Sweeny and Weiner,[73,74] McMahon et al.,[75] Chengelis,[76] and Santa Maria and Machado[77] showed hepatic UGT activity toward acetaminophen and p-nitrophenol was decreased in senescent rats compared to young or adult rats. However, Jayaraj et al.[78] and Borghoff and Birnbaum[79] found no age-related changes in UGT activity toward p-nitrophenol in male Fisher 344 rats after 4 months of age. Such discrepancies may be due partly to the test substrate for UGT; for example, Handler and Brian[80] reported unchanged glucuronidation of p-nitrophenol in livers of young and senescent rats, while glucuronidation of p-nitrocatechol (a hydroxylated p-nitrophenol) was decreased in older rats. Further, UGT activity toward estrone was increased with age, while activity toward testosterone, morphine, and naphthol remained constant.[81,82] The impact of age on UGT glucuronidation of flavonoids has not been investigated.

UDP-glucuronic acid generated from the UDP-glucose dehydrogenase is a major determinant of the rate of UGT-catalyzed glucuronidation.[83] Thus, an age-dependent decrease in UDP-glucose dehydrogenase could limit UDP-GA availability and subsequently decrease the capacity for glucuronidation.[77] Before excretion, glucuronide conjugates of xenobiotics can be cleaved by β-glucuronidase in lysosomes and microsomes.[19] An age-related increase in β-glucuronidase activity reported in rats[79] could enhance the turnover flavonoid–glucuronide conjugates and decrease their rate of excretion. While it is feasible that age-related decreases in UGT activity and UDP-glucuronic acid content and increases in β-glucuronidase activity could impact flavonoid metabolism, studies are required to demonstrate such changes.

In addition to glucuronidation, flavonoids are conjugated with sulfate via SULT, although sulfation reactions are less prevalent due to the limited availability of inorganic sulfate.[84] Using paracetamol as substrate, Herd et al.[71] found human hepatic SULT activity *in vitro* was unaltered by age. However, using p-nitrophenol, Sweeny and Weiner[74] and Galinsky et al.[81] showed hepatic sulfation was lower in senescent male Fisher 344 rats compared with young adults. Galinsky et al.[81] reported a smaller reduction in SULT activity toward acetaminophen or glycolithocholate than toward p-nitrophenol in Fisher rats. Thus, similar to UGT, the age-associated decline in SULT activity appears substrate specific.

COMT-catalyzed reactions with flavonoids do not yield metabolites with increased polarity or water solubility, but these methylated products may be important bioactive forms. Information on age-related changes in COMT is limited. Lee et al.[85] and Stramentinoli et al.[86] found COMT activity in rats was enhanced with age. In contrast, mRNA expression of COMT was 1.3-fold lower in 26- than 3-mo-old male C3H/a mice.[87] Given the potential bioactivation of flavonoids by COMT, characterizing age-related changes in this enzyme is warranted.

Changes in capacity of phase II metabolism across the life span, particularly during advanced ages, appear dependent on both the xenobiotic substrate and the test model, including species and strain of animal.[73] In this regard, the absence of relevant data on flavonoids presents a large gap in the knowledge base of these phytochemicals. Interestingly, Rumore and Blaiklock[88] found young children excreted 50% of acetaminophen as a sulfate conjugate but adults excreted 55% as a glucuronide. As many flavonoids are metabolized by phase II enzymes, their impact on health outcomes may be significantly affected by such age-related changes in metabolism. As even basic information is absent in this area, it is not possible to consider the impact of recently characterized polymorphisms in these enzymes.[89,90]

Effect of Flavonoids on Phase II Metabolism

Flavonoid intake affects phase I and II metabolism and thereby, after chronic consumption, modifies its own bioavailability and kinetics. For example, Kim et al.[91] observed that maximum catechin concentrations in rat blood and tissues were achieved after intake of green tea for 2 days but that, after 28 days of continued consumption, concentrations fell to those found at day 1. Similarly, Manach et al.[92] found the overall bioavailability of quercetin was smaller in rats adapted to a quercetin diet than in nonadapted rats and also showed different metabolite profiles. This indication of the modulation of phase II metabolism by flavonoids is illustrated in the up-regulation of rat hepatic and intestinal UGT activity toward p-nitrophenol by a 2-week dietary intervention with 1% quercetin.[93] Similarly, Petri et al.[94] reported that an acute intake of quercetin led to a 2.4-fold induction of UDP-glucuronosyl transferase 1A1 (UGT1A1) mRNA in exfoliated human enterocytes. In contrast, Canivenc-Lavier et al.[95] found no effect on rat hepatic UGT activity toward p-nitrophenol after supplementation for 2 weeks with 0.3% quercetin. However, this discrepancy may be due to different intakes of dietary quercetin and/or other differences in experimental design (e.g., use of food deprivation[96] and potential differential phase II induction among organs).[64,69] UGT up-regulation is substrate specific; for example, Bu-Abbas et al.[97] found chronic catechin-rich green tea consumption for 4 weeks enhanced hepatic UGT activity toward 2-aminophenol by 100% in rats but found no change toward methylumbelliferone.

Although quercetin may stimulate UGT, it inhibits human hepatic sulfation of resveratrol, acetaminophen, dopamine, (–)-salbutamol, minoxidil, and paracetamol in vitro.[69,98–101] This inhibition may be chemopreventive, as activation of some promutagens occurs via SULT reactions.[68] However, SULT inhibition may also lead to the accumulation of some xenobiotics and possible toxicity. The magnitude of inhibition by quercetin of SULT appears dependent on the isoform because SULT1A3 is less affected than other isoforms, suggesting a tissue-dependent effect of quercetin.[69]

COMT methylates quercetin to form isorhamnetin and tamarixetin, but quercetin can inhibit COMT methylation of catechol estrogens in human liver and mammary cells[102,103] as well as hamster liver and kidney cells.[104] In contrast to an acute dose, consumption of quercetin for 10 days by rats altered the position of methylation, as tamarixetin was undetected in the circulation.[92]

Although flavonoids can modulate UGT, SULT, and COMT activity toward other xenobiotics, their impact after chronic consumption on their own metabolism has not been examined, even though such activity could substantially alter their bioactivity.[105–107] This relationship may become even more complex in older subjects due to the inverse association between age and the adaptability of phase II metabolism.[42,108]

Interactions between Phytochemicals and Phase II Metabolism

All dietary guidelines encourage the consumption of a diverse array of fruits and vegetables. However, relatively little is known about the impact of mixed foods on the bioavailability of phytochemicals.[25,26,30,109,110] For example, Silberberg et al.[27] found that chronic co-administration of quercetin and catechin to rats decreased quercetin absorption by 35% compared to consumption of quercetin alone. Further, herbs and spices may affect the metabolism of flavonoids by modulating phase II metabolism. For example, the alkaloid piperine in black pepper reduces the capacity of glucuronidation in rats and guinea pigs by inhibiting UGT activity and decreasing UDP-glucuronic acid[111,112]—effects that could increase flavonoid bioavailability through less glucuronidation. Indeed, Lambert et al.[113] found piperine enhanced epigallocatechin-3-gallate bioavailability from green tea, possibly by inhibiting intestinal but not hepatic glucuronidation. Shoba et al.[114] also found piperine augmented the bioavailability and serum concentration of curcumin in rats and humans. An increase in methylated epigallocatechin-3-gallate in HT-29 found in human colon cancer cells treated with piperine suggests enhanced COMT activity by piperine.[113]

However, the effect of piperine on SULT and flavonoid status across the life cycle remains to be investigated. Induction of phase II metabolism appears to decrease the bioavailability and accelerate the excretion of flavonoids. For example, Siess et al.[115] and Walle et al.[116] reported flavones induced rat hepatic UGT activity in HepG2 and Caco-2 cells. This induction of UGT enhanced quercetin glucuronidation in Caco-2 cells. In addition to inducing UGT activity, the flavone chrysin inhibits hepatic SULT-mediated sulfation of acetaminophen and minoxidol.[99] The impact of chrysin on the capacity of COMT action toward flavonoids has not been examined. Further, the effect of age on phase II modulation by piperine and chrysin has not been reported. Thus, information on the relationship between age and intake of flavonoids and other phytochemicals that also affect phase II metabolism is required.

EVIDENCE OF AN IMPACT OF AGE ON FLAVONOID STATUS

Although evidence of age-related effects on flavonoid bioavailability and pharmacokinetics is scarce, we have observed that age significantly affects plasma and hepatic concentrations of the isoflavone genistein in male Sprague–Dawley rats.[117] Adult (1 year) and senescent (2 years) rats were fed with 154 or 308 ppm genistein for 5 weeks. After a 12-hour fast, the senescent rats consistently maintained a lower steady state of genistein in plasma than the adult rats, despite similar genistein intakes (Figure 2.4). Aging also decreased genistein concentrations in the liver, though not in the gastrocnemius muscle. Interestingly, Skrzydlewska et al.[118] reported that catechin concentrations in the brain are inversely associated with age in rats fed green tea plus ethanol for 4 weeks. These data suggest age-related changes in flavonoid status, though the underlying mechanisms for this relationship have not been determined.

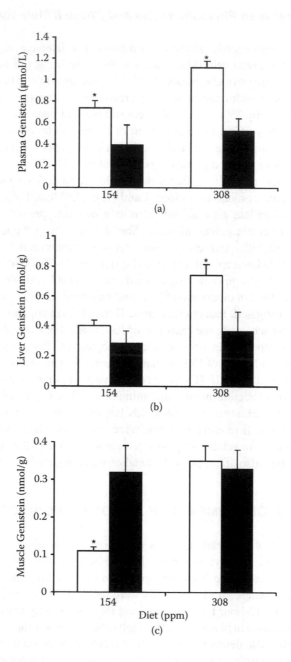

Figure 2.4 Plasma and liver genistein concentration in adult (1 year) and senescent (2 years) Sprague–Dawley rats fed 154 and 308 ppm genistein for 5 wk. Values are means ± SEM, n = 6 in the adult group (white bar) and = 4 in the senescent group (black bar). *Values in the same diet differ, $P \leq 0.05$.

CONCLUSION

The risk of chronic disease associated with aging is largely the result of a progressive loss of physiological and physical functions and reserves and impaired adaptive mechanisms to environmental and endogenous stresses.[119,120] It is also evident that environmental factors, including diets characterized by generous intakes of flavonoid-rich plant foods and low in saturated and *trans*-fatty acids, can reduce the risk of the most prevalent chronic diseases. However, the knowledge base of the bioavailability and metabolism of flavonoids and related polyphenols across the life cycle is scarce and limits our ability to provide quantitative dietary recommendations about foods containing these phytochemicals. Few data are available to inform the rational design of a clinical trial examining the effect of flavonoids on the risk of chronic disease. It is also worth noting that research studies rarely employ older adults, despite this group being a critical target group for health promotion. Therefore, definitive studies characterizing flavonoid bioavailability, metabolism, and distribution across the life cycle—especially in older people—are warranted and will contribute to better substantiated nutrient allowances and dietary guidelines.

ACKNOWLEDGMENT

Support for this work was provided by the U.S. Department of Agriculture (USDA) Agricultural Research Service under Cooperative Agreement No. 58-1950-4-401. The content of this publication does not necessarily reflect the views or policies of the USDA, and does not mention of trade names, commercial products, or organizations imply endorsement by the U.S. government.

REFERENCES

1. Arts, I.C. et al., Catechin intake might explain the inverse relation between tea consumption and ischemic heart disease: The Zutphen Elderly Study, *Am. J. Clin. Nutr.*, 74, 227, 2001.
2. Hertog, M.G. et al., Dietary antioxidant flavonoids and risk of coronary heart disease: The Zutphen Elderly Study, *Lancet*, 342, 1007, 1993.
3. Huxley, R.R. and Neil, H.A., The relation between dietary flavonol intake and coronary heart disease mortality: A meta-analysis of prospective cohort studies, *Eur. J. Clin. Nutr.*, 57, 904, 2003.
4. Jiang, R. et al., Nut and peanut butter consumption and risk of type 2 diabetes in women, *JAMA*, 288, 2554, 2002.
5. Tobias, M. et al., Vegetable and fruit intake and mortality from chronic disease in New Zealand, *Aust. N.Z. J. Public Health*, 30, 26, 2006.
6. Liu, R.H., Potential synergy of phytochemicals in cancer prevention: Mechanism of action, *J. Nutr.*, 134, 3479S, 2004.
7. Treutter, D., Significance of flavonoids in plant resistance and enhancement of their biosynthesis, *Plant Biol. (Stuttg.)*, 7, 581, 2005.

8. Keli, S.O. et al., Dietary flavonoids, antioxidant vitamins, and incidence of stroke: The Zutphen study, *Arch. Intern. Med.*, 156, 637, 1996.
9. Geleijnse, J.M. et al., Tea flavonoids may protect against atherosclerosis: The Rotterdam Study, *Arch. Intern. Med.*, 159, 2170, 1999.
10. Yochum, L. et al., Dietary flavonoid intake and risk of cardiovascular disease in postmenopausal women, *Am. J. Epidemiol.*, 49, 943, 1999.
11. Aherne, S.A. and O'Brien, N.M., Dietary flavonols: Chemistry, food content, and metabolism, *Nutrition*, 18, 75, 2002.
12. Manach, C. et al., Polyphenols: Food sources and bioavailability, *Am. J. Clin. Nutr.*, 79, 727, 2004.
13. Bravo, L., Polyphenols: Chemistry, dietary sources, metabolism, and nutritional significance, *Nutr. Rev.*, 56, 317, 1998.
14. Mink, P.J. et al., Flavonoid intake and cardiovascular disease mortality: A prospective study in postmenopausal women, *Am. J. Clin. Nutr.*, 85, 895, 2007.
15. Manach, C. et al., Bioavailability and bioefficacy of polyphenols in humans I. Review of 97 bioavailability studies, *Am. J. Clin. Nutr.*, 81, 230S, 2005.
16. King, A. and Young, G., Characteristics and occurrence of phenolic phytochemicals, *J. Am. Diet. Assoc.*, 99, 213, 1999.
17. Scalbert, A. and Williamson, G., Dietary intake and bioavailability of polyphenols, *J. Nutr.*, 130, 2073S, 2000.
18. Walle, T., Absorption and metabolism of flavonoids, *Free Radic. Biol. Med.*, 36, 829, 2004.
19. O'Leary, K.A. et al., Metabolism of quercetin-7- and quercetin-3-glucuronides by an *in vitro* hepatic model: The role of human beta-glucuronidase, sulfotransferase, catechol-O-methyltransferase and multiresistant protein 2 (MRP2) in flavonoid metabolism, *Biochem. Pharmacol.*, 65, 479, 2003.
20. O'Leary, K.A. et al., Flavonoid glucuronides are substrates for human liver beta-glucuronidase, *FEBS Lett.*, 503, 103, 2001.
21. Chen, C.Y. et al., Flavonoids from almond skins are bioavailable and act synergistically with vitamins C and E to enhance hamster and human LDL resistance to oxidation, *J. Nutr.*, 135, 1366, 2005.
22. Erlund, I. et al., Pharmacokinetics of quercetin from quercetin aglycone and rutin in healthy volunteers, *Eur. J. Clin. Pharmacol.*, 56, 545, 2000.
23. Conquer, J.A. et al., Supplementation with quercetin markedly increases plasma quercetin concentration without effect on selected risk factors for heart disease in healthy subjects, *J. Nutr.*, 128, 593, 1998.
24. Moon, J.H. et al., Accumulation of quercetin conjugates in blood plasma after the short-term ingestion of onion by women, *Am. J. Physiol. Regul. Integr. Comp. Physiol.*, 279, R461, 2000.
25. Cermak, R., Landgraf, S., and Wolffram, S., The bioavailability of quercetin in pigs depends on the glycoside moiety and on dietary factors, *J. Nutr.*, 133, 2802, 2003.
26. Lesser, S., Cermak, R., and Wolffram, S., Bioavailability of quercetin in pigs is influenced by the dietary fat content, *J. Nutr.*, 134, 1508, 2004.
27. Silberberg, M. et al., Co-administration of quercetin and catechin in rats alters their absorption but not their metabolism, *Life Sci.*, 77, 3156, 2005.
28. Blumberg, J., Nutritional needs of seniors, *J. Am. Coll. Nutr.*, 16, 517, 1997.
29. Chernoff, R., Micronutrient requirements in older women, *Am. J. Clin. Nutr.*, 81, 1240S, 2005.
30. Herrlinger, C. and Klotz, U., Drug metabolism and drug interactions in the elderly, *Best Pract. Res. Clin. Gastroenterol.*, 15, 897, 2001.

31. Anantharaju, A., Feller, A., and Chedid, A., Aging liver. A review, *Gerontology*, 48, 343, 2002.
32. Crome, P., What's different about older people, *Toxicology*, 192, 49, 2003.
33. Jensen, G.L., McGee, M., and Binkley, J., Nutrition in the elderly, *Gastroenterol. Clin. North Am.*, 30, 313, 2001.
34. Tregaskis, B.F. and Stevenson, L.H., Pharmacokinetics in old age, *Br. Med. Bull.*, 46, 9, 1990.
35. Williams, L. and Lowenthal, D.T., Drug therapy in the elderly, *South Med. J.*, 85, 127, 1992.
36. Cohn, S.H. et al., Compartmental body composition based on total-body nitrogen, potassium, and calcium, *Am. J. Physiol.*, 239, E524, 1980.
37. Cusack, B.J., Pharmacokinetics in older persons, *Am. J. Geriatr. Pharmacother.*, 2, 274, 2004.
38. Jensen, G.L. and Rogers, J., Obesity in older persons, *J. Am. Diet. Assoc.*, 98, 1308, 1998.
39. Uauy, R. et al., The changing pattern of whole body protein metabolism in aging humans, *J. Gerontol.*, 33, 663, 1978.
40. Turnheim, K., Drug dosage in the elderly. Is it rational? *Drugs Aging*, 13, 357, 1998.
41. Boulton, D.W., Walle, U.K., and Walle, T., Extensive binding of the bioflavonoid quercetin to human plasma proteins, *J. Pharm. Pharmacol.*, 50, 243, 1998.
42. Iber, F.L., Murphy, P.A., and Connor, E.S., Age-related changes in the gastrointestinal system. Effects on drug therapy, *Drugs Aging*, 5, 34, 1994.
43. Greenblatt, D.J., Reduced serum albumin concentration in the elderly: A report from the Boston Collaborative Drug Surveillance Program, *J. Am. Geriatr. Soc.*, 27, 20, 1979.
44. Campion, E.W., deLabry, L.O., and Glynn, R.J., The effect of age on serum albumin in healthy males: Report from the Normative Aging Study, *J. Gerontol.*, 43, M18, 1988.
45. Foligne, B. et al., Trophic status of the small intestine in young and aged rats: Modulation by a yogurt-supplemented diet, *Dig. Dis. Sci.*, 49, 1291, 2004.
46. Hohn, P., Gabbert, H., and Wagner, R., Differentiation and aging of the rat intestinal mucosa. II. Morphological, enzyme histochemical and disc electrophoretic aspects of the aging of the small intestinal mucosa, *Mech. Ageing Dev.*, 7, 217, 1978.
47. Holt, P.R., Tierney, A.R., and Kotler, D.P., Delayed enzyme expression: A defect of aging rat gut, *Gastroenterology*, 89, 1026, 1985.
48. Majumdar, A.P., Jaszewski, R., and Dubick, M.A., Effect of aging on the gastrointestinal tract and the pancreas, *Proc. Soc. Exp. Biol. Med.*, 215, 134, 1997.
49. Orr, W.C. and Chen, C.L., Aging and neural control of the GI tract: IV. Clinical and physiological aspects of gastrointestinal motility and aging, *Am. J. Physiol. Gastrointest. Liver. Physiol.*, 283, G1226, 2002.
50. Saltzman, J.R. and Russell, R.M., The aging gut. Nutritional issues, *Gastroenterol. Clin. North Am.*, 27, 309, 1998.
51. Wiley, J.W., Aging and neural control of the GI tract: III. Senescent enteric nervous system: Lessons from extraintestinal sites and nonmammalian species, *Am. J. Physiol. Gastrointest. Liver Physiol.*, 283, G1020, 2002.
52. McLean, A.J. and Le Couteur, D.G., Aging biology and geriatric clinical pharmacology, *Pharmacol. Rev.*, 56, 163, 2004.
53. Woodhouse, K. and Wynne, H.A., Age-related changes in hepatic function. Implications for drug therapy, *Drugs Aging*, 2, 243, 1992.
54. Wallis, J.L. et al., Duodenal brush-border mucosal glucose transport and enzyme activities in aging man and effect of bacterial contamination of the small intestine, *Dig. Dis. Sci.*, 38, 403, 1993.

34   C-Y. OLIVER CHEN AND JEFFREY B. BLUMBERG

55. Lee, M.F. et al., Total intestinal lactase and sucrase activities are reduced in aged rats, *J. Nutr.*, 127, 1382, 1997.
56. Lipski, P.S. et al., Ageing and duodenal morphometry, *J. Clin. Pathol.*, 45, 450, 1992.
57. Wynne, H., Drug metabolism and ageing, *J. Br. Menopause. Soc.*, 11, 51, 2005.
58. Woodhouse, K.W. and Wynne, H.A., Age-related changes in liver size and hepatic blood flow. The influence on drug metabolism in the elderly, *Clin. Pharmacokinet.*, 15, 287, 1988.
59. Wynne, H.A. et al., The effect of age and frailty upon acetanilide clearance in man, *Age Ageing*, 18, 415, 1989.
60. Wynne, H.A. et al., Hepatic drug clearance: The effect of age using indocyanine green as a model compound, *Br. J. Clin. Pharmacol.*, 30, 634, 1990.
61. Zeeh. J. and Platt, D., The aging liver: Structural and functional changes and their consequences for drug treatment in old age, *Gerontology*, 48, 121, 2002.
62. Birnbaum, L.S., Pharmacokinetic basis of age-related changes in sensitivity to toxicants, *Annu. Rev. Pharmacol. Toxicol.*, 31, 101, 1991.
63. Rikans, L.E., Influence of aging on chemically induced hepatotoxicity: Role of age-related changes in metabolism, *Drug Metab. Rev.*, 20, 87, 1989.
64. Glatt, H. and Meinl, W., Pharmacogenetics of soluble sulfotransferases (SULTs), *Naunyn Schmiedebergs Arch. Pharmacol.*, 369, 55, 2004.
65. Mackenzie, P.I. et al., The UDP glycosyltransferase gene superfamily: Recommended nomenclature update based on evolutionary divergence, *Pharmacogenetics*, 7, 255, 1997.
66. Tukey, R.H. and Strassburg, C.P., Human UDP-glucuronosyltransferases: Metabolism, expression, and disease, *Annu. Rev. Pharmacol. Toxicol.*, 40, 581, 2000.
67. King, C. et al., Characterization of rat and human UDP-glucuronosyltransferases responsible for the *in vitro* glucuronidation of diclofenac, *Toxicol. Sci.*, 61, 49, 2001.
68. Wang, L.Q. and James, M.O., Inhibition of sulfotransferases by xenobiotics, *Curr. Drug. Metab.*, 7, 83, 2006.
69. Marchetti, F. et al., Differential inhibition of human liver and duodenum sulphotransferase activities by quercetin, a flavonoid present in vegetables, fruit and wine, *Xenobiotica*, 31, 841, 2001.
70. Zhu, B.T., Catechol-O-Methyltransferase (COMT)-mediated methylation metabolism of endogenous bioactive catechols and modulation by endobiotics and xenobiotics: Importance in pathophysiology and pathogenesis, *Curr. Drug Metab.*, 3, 321, 2002.
71. Herd, B. et al., The effect of age on glucuronidation and sulphation of paracetamol by human liver fractions, *Br. J. Clin. Pharmacol.*, 32, 768, 1991.
72. Hansen, K.T. and Stentoft, K., Characterization of benzazepine UDP-glucuronosyl-transferases in laboratory animals and man, *Xenobiotica*, 25, 611, 1995.
73. Sweeny, D.J. and Weiner, M., Metabolism of acetaminophen in hepatocytes isolated from mice and rats of various ages, *Drug Metab. Dispos.*, 13, 377, 1985.
74. Sweeny, D.J. and Weiner, M., Effect of aging on the metabolism of *p*-nitroanisole and *p*-nitrophenol in isolated hepatocytes, *Age*, 9, 95, 1985.
75. McMahon, T.F., Beierschmitt, W.P., and Weiner, M., Changes in phase I and phase II biotransformation with age in male Fischer 344 rat colon: Relationship to colon carcinogenesis, *Cancer Lett.*, 36, 273, 1987.
76. Chengelis, C.P., Age- and sex-related changes in epoxide hydrolase, UDP-glucuronosyl transferase, glutathione S-transferase, and PAPS sulphotransferase in Sprague–Dawley rats, *Xenobiotica*, 18, 1225, 1988.

77. Santa Maria, C. and Machado, A., Changes in some hepatic enzyme activities related to phase II drug metabolism in male and female rats as a function of age, *Mech. Ageing Dev.*, 44, 115, 1988.

78. Jayaraj, A. et al., Metabolism, covalent binding, and mutagenicity of aflatoxin B1 by liver extracts from rats of various ages, *J. Natl. Cancer Inst.*, 74, 95, 1985.

79. Borghoff, S.J. and Birnbaum, L.S., Age-related changes in glucuronidation and deglucuronidation in liver, small intestine, lung, and kidney of male Fischer rats, *Drug Metab. Dispos.*, 13, 62, 1985.

80. Handler, J.A. and Brian, W.R., Effect of aging on mixed-function oxidation and conjugation by isolated perfused rat livers, *Biochem. Pharmacol.*, 54, 159, 1997.

81. Galinsky, R.E. et al., Effect of aging on hepatic biotransformation in female Fischer 344 rats: Changes in sulfotransferase activities are consistent with known gender-related changes in pituitary growth hormone secretion in aging animals, *J. Pharmacol. Exp. Ther.*, 255, 577, 1990.

82. Galinsky, R.E., Kane, R.E., and Franklin, M.R., Effect of aging on drug-metabolizing enzymes important in acetaminophen elimination, *J. Pharmacol. Exp. Ther.*, 237, 107, 1986.

83. Reinke, L.A. et al., Conjugation of *p*-nitrophenol in the perfused rat liver: The effect of substrate concentration and carbohydrate reserves, *J. Pharmacol. Exp. Ther.*, 217, 863, 1981.

84. Sheweita, S.A., Drug-metabolizing enzymes: Mechanisms and functions, *Curr. Drug Metab.*, 1, 107, 2000.

85. Lee, J.J. et al., Changes in endogenous monoamines in aged rats, *Clin. Exp. Pharmacol. Physiol.*, 28, 285, 2001.

86. Stramentinoli, G. et al., Tissue levels of S-adenosylmethionine in aging rats, *J. Gerontol.*, 32, 392, 1977.

87. Mikhailova, O.N., Gulyaeva, L.F., and Filipenko, M.L., Gene expression of drug metabolizing enzymes in adult and aged mouse liver: A modulation by immobilization stress, *Toxicology*, 210, 189, 2005.

88. Rumore, M.M. and Blaiklock, R.G., Influence of age-dependent pharmacokinetics and metabolism on acetaminophen hepatotoxicity, *J. Pharm. Sci.*, 81, 203, 1992.

89. Dorne, J.L., Impact of interindividual differences in drug metabolism and pharmacokinetics on safety evaluation, *Fundam. Clin. Pharmacol.*, 18, 609, 2004.

90. Miners, J.O., McKinnon, R.A., and Mackenzie, P.I., Genetic polymorphisms of UDP-glucuronosyltransferases and their functional significance, *Toxicology*, 181–182, 453, 2002.

91. Kim, S. et al., Plasma and tissue levels of tea catechins in rats and mice during chronic consumption of green tea polyphenols, *Nutr. Cancer*, 37, 41, 2000.

92. Manach, C. et al., Bioavailability of rutin and quercetin in rats, *FEBS Lett.*, 409, 12, 1997.

93. van der Logt, E.M. et al., Induction of rat hepatic and intestinal UDP-glucuronosyltransferases by naturally occurring dietary anticarcinogens, *Carcinogenesis*, 24, 1651, 2003.

94. Petri, N. et al., Absorption/metabolism of sulforaphane and quercetin, and regulation of phase II enzymes, in human jejunum *in vivo*, *Drug Metab. Dispos.*, 31, 805, 2003.

95. Canivenc-Lavier, M.C. et al., Comparative effects of flavonoids and model inducers on drug-metabolizing enzymes in rat liver, *Toxicology*, 114, 19, 1996.

96. Siegers, C.P., Bartels, L., and Riemann, D., Effects of fasting and glutathione depletors on the GSH-dependent enzyme system in the gastrointestinal mucosa of the rat, *Pharmacology*, 38, 121, 1989.

97. Bu-Abbas, A. et al., Stimulation of rat hepatic UDP-glucuronosyl transferase activity following treatment with green tea, *Food Chem. Toxicol.*, 33, 27, 1995.
98. De Santi, C. et al., Sulphation of resveratrol, a natural compound present in wine, and its inhibition by natural flavonoids, *Xenobiotica*, 30, 857, 2000.
99. Eaton, E.A. et al., Flavonoids, potent inhibitors of the human P-form phenolsulfotransferase. Potential role in drug metabolism and chemoprevention, *Drug Metab. Dispos.*, 24, 232, 1996.
100. Ghazali, R.A. and Waring, R.H., The effects of flavonoids on human phenolsulphotransferases: Potential in drug metabolism and chemoprevention, *Life Sci.*, 65, 1625, 1999.
101. Mesia-Vela, S. and Kauffman, F.C., Inhibition of rat liver sulfotransferases SULT1A1 and SULT2A1 and glucuronosyltransferase by dietary flavonoids, *Xenobiotica*, 33, 1211, 2003.
102. Nagai, M., Conney, A.H., and Zhu, B.T., Strong inhibitory effects of common tea catechins and bioflavonoids on the O-methylation of catechol estrogens catalyzed by human liver cytosolic catechol-O-methyltransferase, *Drug Metab. Dispos.*, 32, 497, 2004.
103. van Duursen, M.B. et al., Phytochemicals inhibit catechol-O-methyltransferase activity in cytosolic fractions from healthy human mammary tissues: Implications for catechol estrogen-induced DNA damage, *Toxicol. Sci.*, 81, 316, 2004.
104. Zhu, B.T. and Liehr, J.G., Inhibition of catechol O-methyltransferase-catalyzed O-methylation of 2- and 4-hydroxyestradiol by quercetin. Possible role in estradiol-induced tumorigenesis, *J. Biol. Chem.*, 271, 1357, 1996.
105. Hecht, S.S., Chemoprevention of cancer by isothiocyanates, modifiers of carcinogen metabolism, *J. Nutr.*, 129, 768S, 1999.
106. Kelloff, G.J. et al., Progress in cancer chemoprevention: Development of diet-derived chemopreventive agents, *J. Nutr.*, 130, 467S, 2000.
107. Waladkhani, A.R. and Clemens, M.R., Effect of dietary phytochemicals on cancer development, *Int. J. Mol. Med.*, 1, 747, 1998.
108. Rossi, A.M. et al., Phenotype–genotype relationships of SULT1A1 in human liver and variations in the IC50 of the SULT1A1 inhibitor quercetin, *Int. J. Clin. Pharmacol. Ther.*, 42, 561, 2004.
109. Dragoni, S. et al., Red wine alcohol promotes quercetin absorption and directs its metabolism towards isorhamnetin and tamarixetin in rat intestine *in vitro*, *Br. J. Pharmacol.*, 147, 765–771, 2006.
110. Kobayashi, Y. et al., Green tea polyphenols inhibit the sodium-dependent glucose transporter of intestinal epithelial cells by a competitive mechanism, *J. Agric. Food Chem.*, 48, 5618, 2000.
111. Reen, R.K. et al., Impairment of UDP-glucose dehydrogenase and glucuronidation activities in liver and small intestine of rat and guinea pig *in vitro* by piperine, *Biochem. Pharmacol.*, 46, 229, 1993.
112. Singh, J., Dubey, R.K., and Atal, C.K., Piperine-mediated inhibition of glucuronidation activity in isolated epithelial cells of the guinea-pig small intestine: Evidence that piperine lowers the endogeneous UDP-glucuronic acid content, *J. Pharmacol. Exp. Ther.*, 236, 488, 1986.
113. Lambert, J.D. et al., Piperine enhances the bioavailability of the tea polyphenol (−)-epigallo-catechin-3-gallate in mice, *J. Nutr.*, 134, 1948, 2004.
114. Shoba, G. et al., Influence of piperine on the pharmacokinetics of curcumin in animals and human volunteers, *Planta Med.*, 64, 353, 1998.
115. Siess, M.H. et al., Time course of induction of rat hepatic drug-metabolizing enzyme activities following dietary administration of flavonoids, *J. Toxicol. Environ. Health*, 49, 481, 1996.

116. Walle, T. et al., Induction of UDP-glucuronosyltransferase UGT1A1 by the flavonoid chrysin in the human hepatoma cell line hep G2, *Drug Metab. Dispos.*, 28, 1077, 2000.
117. Chen, C.Y. and Bakhiet, R.M., Age decreased steady-state concentrations of genistein in plasma, liver, and skeletal muscle in Sprague–Dawley rats, *Mech. Ageing Dev.*, 127, 344, 2006.
118. Skrzydlewska, E. et al., Green tea supplementation in rats of different ages mitigates ethanol-induced changes in brain antioxidant abilities, *Alcohol*, 37, 89, 2005.
119. Grimley Evans, J., Twenty-first century: Review: Ageing and medicine, *J. Intern. Med.*, 247, 159, 2000.
120. Kirkwood, T.B. and Austad, S.N., Why do we age? *Nature*, 408, 233, 2000.

CHAPTER 3

Trends in the Analysis of Phytochemicals
Flavonoids and Carotenoids

Eunmi Koh and Alyson E. Mitchell

CONTENTS

INTRODUCTION

Polyphenols and carotenoids are naturally occurring phytochemicals found in plants. Recent epidemiological evidence suggests that numerous polyphenols and carotenoids have health-promoting properties that may reduce the risk associated with chronic diseases such as cardiovascular disease and certain cancers.[64,78] Polyphenols represent a class of secondary plant metabolites (SPMs) that play critical roles in the physiology of plants, including pigmentation, resistance to pathogen stress and herbivory, and protection against ultraviolet (UV)-B radiation.[27,50] The polyphenolic profiles of plants differ between species and varieties of the same species and are generally synthesized in response to environmental pressures.

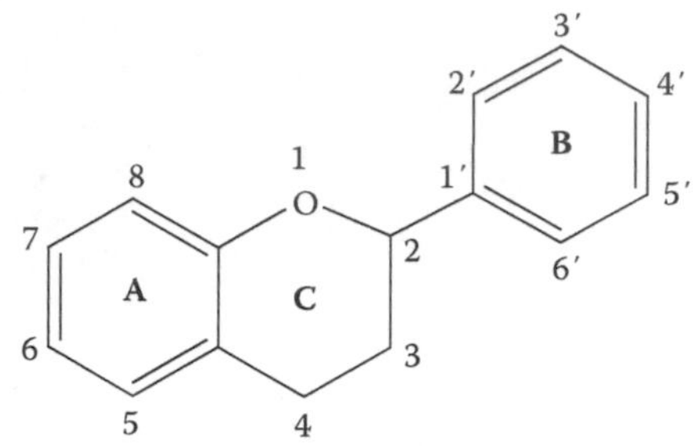

Figure 3.1   The structure of the C_6-C_3-C_6 flavan nucleus.

Flavonoids represent the most common and widely distributed class of polyphenolics in the Western diet. To date, about 6500 flavonoids have been identified.[50] All are phenylpropanoid derivatives based on the C_6-C_3-C_6 flavan nucleus (Figure 3.1). Flavonoids can be placed into subclasses based upon the degree of saturation and oxidation present in the heterocyclic ring (C-ring) of the flavan nucleus. Subclasses include the flavones, flavonols, flavanones, flavan-3-ols, anthocyanins, and isoflavones (Table 3.1). Isoflavones differ from the other flavonoid subclasses, as they have the B-ring attached to the C-3 of the heterocyclic C-ring. Flavonoids occur as *O*-glycosides or, less frequently, *C*-glycosides, although aglycones are sometimes found in edible plants as well (e.g., the catechin and epicatechin aglycones present in cocoa). The sugars of the *O*-glycosides are generally bound to the hydroxyl groups of the flavonoid nucleus at at C-3 and/or C-7 positions, whereas *C*-glycosides are attached to either the C-6 or C-8 positions. Unlike the *O*-glycosides, the *C*-glycosides are not cleaved by acid hydrolysis. In numerous plants, the sugars are often further substituted by acetyl, malonyl, or organic acid residues (e.g., the isoflavones in soybeans and anthocyanidins in wine).

Carotenoids are a class of fat-soluble, light-harvesting pigments found in plants; however, they are also found in some algae, photosynthetic bacteria, yeasts, and molds. Carotenoids play a critical role in photosynthesis by protecting the photosynthetic apparatus from damage associated with the production of chlorophyll triplet states and singlet oxygen. Carotenoids are responsible for many of the red, orange, and yellow hues of fruits, flowers, and leaves as well as the colors of some birds, fish, and crustaceans. Carotenoids are derived from a 40-carbon polyene chain. This chain may be linear or terminated by cyclic end-groups and may contain oxygen-containing functional groups (Figure 3.2). Carotenoids composed of only carbon and hydrogen are called carotenes and include lycopene, β-carotene, and α-carotene. Oxygenated derivatives are called xanthophylls and include zeaxanthin, lutein, violaxanthin, β-cryptoxanthin, and capsanthin. About 600 carotenoids have been identified to date.[91] The conjugated double bonds common to all carotenoids are present primarily in the more thermodynamically stable *trans* configuration; however, these bonds can be isomerized to the *cis* configuration in the presence of pro-oxidants, thermal processing, and the exposure to light. Animals lack the ability to synthesize

Table 3.1 Chemical Structures of Flavonoids Found in Plants

Group	Compound	R_1	R_2	R_3	R_4	R_5
Flavonols	Quercetin	OH	OH	H	OH	OH
	Kaempferol	H	OH	H	OH	OH
	Myricetin	OH	OH	OH	OH	OH
	Morin	OH	H	OH	H	OH
	Isorhamnetin	OCH_3	OH	H	OH	OH
	Quercitrin	OH	OH	H	O-rham	OH
	Rutin	OH	OH	H	O-rut	OH
Flavanones	Naringenin	H	OH	OH		
	Naringin	H	OH	O-neo		
	Narirutin	H	OH	O-rut		
	Hesperidin	H	OCH_3	O-rut		
	Hesperitin	H	OCH_3	OH		
	Neohesperidin	OH	OCH_3	O-neo		
	Didymin	H	OCH_3	O-rut		
	Prunin	H	OH	O-glu		
Flavan-3-ols	(+)-Catechin	H	OH			
	(–)-Epicatechin	H	OH			
	(–)-Epicatechin gallate	H	O-gall			
	(–)-Epigallocatechin	OH	OH			
	(–)-Epigallocatechin gallate	OH	O-gall			

(continued on next page)

Table 3.1 (continued) Chemical Structures of Flavonoids Found in Plants

Group	Compound	R_1	R_2	R_3	R_4	R_5
Isoflavones	Daidzein	OH	H	OH		
	Daidzin	OH	H	O-glu		
	Genistein	OH	OH	OH		
	Genistin	OH	H	O-glu		
	Formononetin	OCH_3	H	OH		
	Biochanin A	OCH_3	OH	OH		
	Ononin	OCH_3	H	O-glu		
	Sissotrin	OCH_3	OH	O-glu		
Anthocyanins	Pelargonidin	H	OH	H		
	Cyanidin	OH	OH	H		
	Delphinidin	OH	OH	OH		
	Peonidin	OCH_3	OH	H		
	Petunidin	OCH_3	OH	OH		
	Malvidin	OCH_3	OH	OCH3		

Notes: Rham, rhamnose; neo, neohesperidise, rhamnosyl-$(\alpha1\rightarrow2)$-glucoside; rut, rutinoside, rhamnosyl-$(\alpha1\rightarrow6)$-glucoside; gall, gallic acid; glu, glucose; arrows represent a major position of glycosylation.

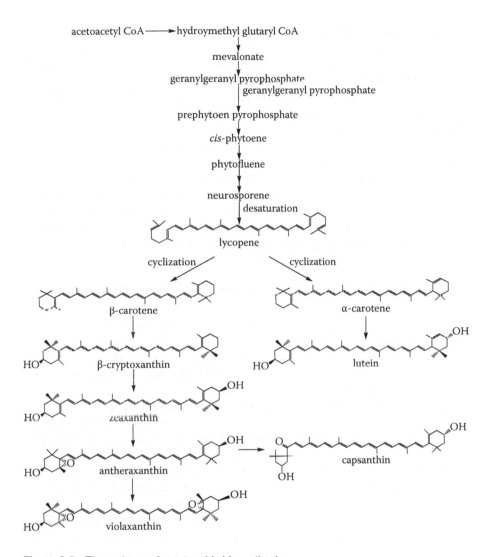

Figure 3.2 The pathway of carotenoids biosynthesis.

carotenoids and require them in the diet (e.g., β-carotene, which is a precursor of vitamin A).

There is a strong epidemiological association between increased fruit and vegetable consumption and the protection against cardiovascular disease[53] and, to a lesser extent, against cancer[64] and other age-related diseases such as dementia.[20] The protection afforded by fruit and vegetables is thought to be due to the complement of antioxidant phytochemicals (e.g., flavonoids, carotenoids, vitamins E and C) along with the minerals and fiber found in these foods. Flavonoids are particularly interesting phytochemicals because not only are they potent *in vitro* antioxidants[29,92] with radical scavenging activity,[108] but they also induce protective enzymes[88] and are thought to play key roles in many of the processes underlying vascular dysfunction and the development of atherosclerosis.[102] Carotenoids are potent *in vitro* antioxidants as well and also demonstrate the ability to delay the onset of arteriosclerosis, cardiovascular disease, and certain types of cancer.[43,89]

It is important to note that although flavonoids and carotenoids are implicated in the prevention of chronic disease, almost all attempts to assign health-promoting activity to the *in vitro* antioxidant action of any one specific compound of these phytochemicals have been unsuccessful. Williamson and Manach[115] point to some of the difficulties in interpreting data from intervention studies of polyphenols, including incomplete characterization of the test material, unvalidated biomarkers, and the lack of understanding of polyphenol bioavailability and metabolism. Recently, themes have shifted away from antioxidant properties of polyphenols and carotenoids toward understanding specific interactions with biomolecules affecting cell signaling, membrane properties, and gene and protein expression.

BIOSYNTHESIS OF FLAVONOIDS AND CAROTENOIDS IN PLANTS

Flavonoids are synthesized in the shikimate and acetate pathways from the basic starting material glucose (Figure 3.3). The A-ring appears to come from resorcinol or phlorogucinol, which is synthesized in the acetate pathway, whereas the B-ring is derived from the shikimate pathway. The shikimate pathways generate the aromatic amino acids phenylalanine, tyrosine, and tryptophan. These are converted into 4-coumaroyl CoA, which is a direct precursor of flavonoids. This intermediate compound condenses with three moles of malonyl-CoA to form naringenin chalcone. Naringenin chalcone is stereospecifically isomerized into naringenin, which is a precursor of the flavonols, flavan-3-ols, procyanidins, and leucoanthocyanidins which are further converted to colored anthocyanidins.[116] A critical regulatory step in the generation of polyphenolics is the deamination of phenylalanine by phenylalanine ammonia lyase (PAL) and subsequent formation of cinnamic acid.

Carotenoids exist primarily with 40 carbon backbones. However, a few bacterial carotenoids containing 30, 45, and 50 carbon atoms have been identified.[41] Carotenoids are synthesized from a five-carbon terpenoid precursor, isopentenyl pyrophosphate (Figure 3.2). Isopentenyl pyrophosphate is converted to geranylgeranyl pyrophosphate (GGPP). The condensation of two molecules of GGPP leads to the eventual formation of phytoene. Phytoene synthesis is the first committed step in C_{40}-carotenoid biosynthesis. This is followed by a stepwise dehydrogenation via phytofluene, ζ-carotene, and neurosporene to give lycopene. Subsequent steps including cyclization, dehydrogenations, and oxidations lead to the range of naturally occurring carotenoids.[26]

The content of flavonoids and carotenoids in plants is influenced by multiple factors, including genotype and environmental conditions. Genotype is regarded as the most influential factor determining the levels of SPMs in crops. Environmental

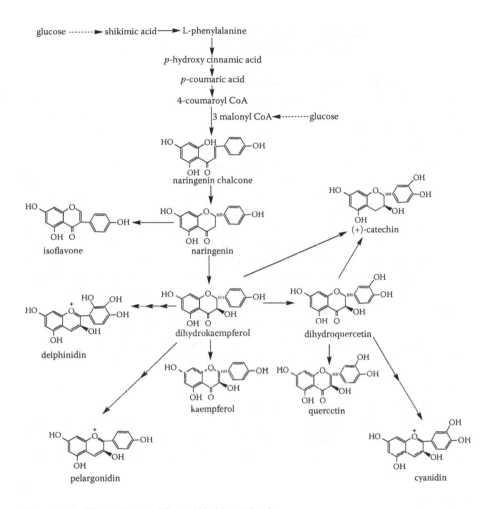

Figure 3.3 The pathway of flavonoids biosynthesis.

stresses such as nutrient deficiency, wounding, pathogens, and UV-B radiation are known to activate the phenylalanine/hydroxycinnamate pathway and subsequently increase the biosynthesis of flavonoids.[27] Additionally, soil quality and type, climate, and water supply affect the levels of flavonoids in plants.[27,50] For example, rapid increases in crop growth and development rates and greater biomass accumulation in well-fertilized crops are thought to have the potential to result in the decreased SPMs.[105] A relationship between decreased nitrogen fertilization and increased flavonoid production was recently demonstrated in a 10-year archive of tomato samples.[85] Temperatures greater than 30°C have also been shown to significantly decrease the lycopene content in tomatoes.[9,106] Interestingly, a recent study by Toor et al.[106] demonstrated that the lycopene content of three tomato cultivars was lower in summer months as compared with spring months.

ANALYSIS OF FLAVONOIDS AND CAROTENOIDS
IN FOODS AND BIOLOGICAL SAMPLES

The accurate measurement of carotenoids and flavonoids in crops and finished foods is becoming increasingly important as the role for these compounds in promoting human health becomes more evident. Reliable and sensitive methods are critical for database development, estimating intake, and assessing the potential health benefits associated with the consumption of specific foods or diets.

Flavonoids and carotenoids encompass broad groups of molecules. They often have very different chemical and physical characteristics within their own class, and require numerous extraction and analytical methods to evaluate their levels in foods. Due to their often complex chemical structures, standards are not always available. This is especially true for some of the more complex glycosidic forms of flavonoids. Over the years, numerous methods have been developed to establish the distribution and content of flavonoids and carotenoids in foods, as well as their metabolites in biological samples. These methods have largely relied on analytical techniques such as the high-performance liquid chromatography (HPLC) and gas chromatography (GC) methods discussed later. Newer techniques such as HPLC interfaced with tandem mass spectrometry (MS/MS) offer the advantage of structural elucidation along with quantification and are also discussed. Numerous factors are now understood to influence the levels of phytochemicals in foods. The primary factors include genotype, plant maturity, plant tissue sampled (i.e., botanical fruit vs. leaf or stem), agronomic practices, environment, microclimate, and pest pressures as well as postharvest storage and processing conditions. These factors were not always appreciated in earlier studies and have led to a large amount of variability in existing data. More recent studies include details regarding these factors and have led to more robust values, which are especially critical for accurate database development and estimating intake.

Flavonoids

Phenolic compounds constitute one of the most numerous and widely distributed groups of phytochemicals in the plant kingdom. More than 8000 phenolic compounds have been described and this list continues to expand.[49] Phenolic compounds exist as simple molecules, such as the phenolic acids, to highly polymerized structures, such as the proanthocyanidins. Harborne[48] classified phenolics into 10 subclasses based upon their chemical structure; these subclasses include the simple phenolics, phenolic acids, hydroxycinnamic acids, and flavonoids, among others. The flavonols represent one of the most commonly distributed classes of flavonoid compounds.

Flavonols

The predominant flavonols found in the Western diet include quercetin (3,3′,4′,5,7-pentahydroxy-2-phenylchromen-4-one), kaempferol(3,4′,5,7-tetrahydroxy-2-phenylchromen-4-one), myricetin (3,3′,4′,5′,5,7-hexahydroxy-2-phenylchromen-

4-one), morin (2-(2,4-dihydroxyphenyl)-3,5,7-trihydroxy-4H-1-benzopyran-4-one), isorhamnetin (3,5,7-trihydroxy-2-(4-hydroxy-3-methoxyphenyl)-4H-chromen-4-one), and their glycosylated forms (Table 3.1). However, of the approximately 380 flavonol glycosides described, the majority are either quercetin or kaempferol derivatives. Common dietary sources of quercetin and kaempferol include onions (340–347 µg quercetin/g fresh weight), kale (110–120 µg quercetin/g and 211–470 µg kaempferol/g fresh weight), and apples (20–36 µg quercetin/g fresh weight).[56] In plants, flavonols are usually found as O-glycosides and C-glycosides, which are characterized by a carbon–carbon linkage between the anomeric carbon of the sugar molecule and either C-6 or C-8 carbon of the flavan nucleus. The O-glycosides occur via a β-glycosidic bond most commonly at 3, 4′, and 7 positions, although the linkage at the C-3 position predominates. Various glycosides, including monosaccharides (quercetin 3-glucoside) and disaccharides (e.g., quercetin 3-rhamnoglucoside, also known as rutin) are common; however, trisaccharides and tetrasaccharides have also been described.[4,77,100,107]

Flavonols are relatively stable compounds that can be extracted from either dried or fresh material (Table 3.2). In general, a polar solvent such as water, aqueous methanol, methanol, or aqueous acetone can be used. Solvent choice will depend upon sample matrix and the solubility characteristics of the individual flavonol glycosides. Alternatively, Hertog et al.[52] described a method for the extraction of flavonol aglycones from several fruits and vegetables via acid hydrolysis using 1.2 M HCl/50% aqueous methanol for 2 hours. This method and several modifications have been used to estimate the levels of total flavonol aglycones in numerous foods and beverages.[25,47,83] Merken et al.[83] described the pseudo first-order kinetic degradation of flavonoids during acid hydrolysis up to 5 hours and pointed to the need to optimize the reaction time and an acid concentration depending on food matrix. Alkaline hydrolysis (0.5% aqueous potassium hydroxide) in a boiling water bath has also been used.[3] In either case, the rate of hydrolysis depends upon the structure of the flavonoid aglycone, the degree of hydroxylation, the position of attachment of the sugar, and the food matrix. After hydrolysis the extracts may contain free sugars, which can be removed by extraction with ethyl acetate or by using solid phase extraction (SPE) on Sephadex, polyamide, or Amberlite. HPLC using UV detection at 360–380 nm is typically used to quantify the levels of total flavonol aglycones.[4,37,77,79,85,90,107]

It is now understood that the glycoside itself influences the bioavailability of flavonols in humans. For example, Hollman et al.[55] demonstrated that quercetin 4′-glucoside was more bioavailable than either the quercetin 3-galactoside or quercetin 3-rutinoside. This observation has increased the need to identify and quantify the levels of individual flavonol glycosides in foods as well as in biological tissues and plasma.[4,37,77,107] Flavonol glycosides are relatively poor chromophores as compared to the parent aglycones; therefore, HPLC methods employing UV detection do not always have the sensitivity and specificity to quantify trace levels of flavonol glycosides or their metabolites, especially in biological fluids. HPLC coupled with diode array detection (DAD) offers the advantage of identifying peaks and determining peak purity, based on characteristic UV-visible spectra in the 200- to 600-nm region. Fluorescent detection can offer an improved sensitivity, but fluorescent derivatives

Table 3.2 Methodological Overview of Flavonol Analysis from Foods and Biological Samples

Sample	Analytes	Sample Preparation	Column	Mobile Phase	Detection	LOD	Ref.
Apple	IS glycosides	Extraction with acetone, centrifugation, acidification, extraction with EtAc	C-18	ACN-H$_2$O-acetic acid	HPLC/DAD/MSn/APCI(−)		100
Broccoli	Glycosides of Q, K, and IS	Freeze-dried, extraction with H$_2$O, SPE with Amberlite and Sephadex, alkaline or acid hydrolysis	C-18	H$_2$O-MeOH-formic acid	HPLC/DAD/MSn/ESI(−)		107
Ginkgo biloba tablet	Q, K, IS, R, QTR	Pulverization, sonication in MeOH, centrifugation	C-18	ACN-H$_2$O-formic acid	HPLC/UV (350 nm)/MS/MS/ESI(−)	R 0.39, Q 1.56, K 1.65, IS 0.38, QTR 0.40 (mg/L)	28
Helleborus atrorubens leaves	Q, K	Air-dried, pulverization, reflux with MeOH, filtration	Silica	EtAc-formic acid-H$_2$O	TLC/UV (366 nm)		79
Herbs	Q, R	Air-dried, pulverization, reflux with MeOH, filtration	Silica	EtOH-borate buffer	CE/ECD	R 0.26, Q 0.07 mg/L	17
Passiflora species leaves	R, IO, O, V	Air-dried, reflux with MeOH, derivatization with diphenylboric acid-2-aminoethylester and PEG 400 in MeOH	Silica	EtAc-formic acid-H$_2$O	HPTLC/densitometry (300 nm)	R 0.46, V 0.42, IO and O 0.47 mg/L	90

Sample	Analytes	Sample preparation	Mobile phase	Method/detection	LOD	Ref.
Sorocea bomplandii leaves	di(tri) glycosides of Q and K	Air-dried, pulverization, boiling in water, SPE with Amberlite XAD-2, ultrasonication, filtration	MeOH-D$_2$O	HPLC/UV(370 nm)/MS/ESI(+), HPLC/NMR		4
Standards	Q, K, IS, M, R, morin	Derivatization with aluminum nitrate reagent	ACN-phosphate buffer	HPLC/FD (485 nm/422 nm)	Q 0.15, K 0.05, M 0.45, IS 0.05 (g/L)	54
Tomato	K-(di)-glycosides, R	Freeze-dried, pulverization, homogenization, extraction with aqueous MeOH, filtration or centrifugation, SPE with polyamide	ACN-H$_2$O-THF-TFA	HPLC/DAD/MS/MS/ESI(+), HPLC/NMR		37
Tomato	Q, K	Air-dried, pulverization, reflux with acidified MeOH, filtration, sonication	ACN-H$_2$O-MeOH-TFA	HPLC/DAD (370 nm)		85
Human plasma, urine	Mono(di) glucuronides of Q and IS	Protein precipitation, centrifugation	ACN-H$_2$O-formic acid	HPLC/DAD (365 nm)/MS/MS/ESI(-)		86
Human and rat serum, plasma, and urine	Q	Extraction with EtAc, centrifugation, derivatization with BSTFA, enzymatic hydrolysis for conjugates	He	GC/MS/SIM	0.01 (g/L)	104

Notes: LOD, limit of detection; Q, quercetin; K, kaempferol; M, myricetin; IS, isorhamnetin; R, rutin; O, orientin; V, vitexin; IO, isoorientin; QTR, quercitrin; MeOH, methanol; EtOH, ethanol; ACN, acetonitrile; EtAc, ethyl acetate; THF, tetrahydrofuran; TFA, trifluoroacetic acid; SPE, solid phase extraction; BSTFA, bis(trimethylsilyl)trifluoroacetamide; GC, gas chromatography; MS, mass spectrometry; HPLC, high-performance liquid chromatography; DAD, diode array detector; FD, fluorescence detector; ESI, electrospray ionization; NMR, nuclear magnetic resonance; APCI, atmospheric pressure chemical ionization; SIM, selected ion monitoring; CE, capillary electrophoresis; ECD, electrochemical detector; TLC, thin layer chromatography; HPTLC, high-performance thin layer chromatography.

and chelates often have to be formed. Flavonols containing a free hydroxyl group at the C-3 position and a keto group at the C-4 position will form fluorescent chelates with various metal ions. For example, Hollman et al.[54] developed a fluorescence method employing postcolumn derivatization of quercetin with Al^{3+}. As compared with UV detection, the sensitivity was 300-fold higher and was reproducible with a relative standard deviation of 1.4%.

LC/MS/MS or HPLC with nuclear magnetic resonance (NMR) methods have also been used to identify unknown flavonol glycosides and their metabolites as reference standards are often not available. For extraction, nonacidic methanol is recommended to avoid acid-catalyzed hydrolysis of β-glycosidic linkages. LC/MS[n] is particularly useful, as it allows the differentiation of sugars attached to aglycones as well as the type of glycosylation (e.g., O-glycosylation or C-glycosylation).[100] In general, negative mode electrospray ionization [ESI(-)/MS/MS] tends to be about 10-fold more sensitive than positive mode ionization [ESI(+)/MS/MS]. Rauha et al.[95] compared the ionization efficiency of five flavonoids, including isorhamnetin, using ESI, atmospheric pressure chemical ionization (APCI), and atmospheric pressure photoionization (APPI) with nine different mobile phase compositions. They found that optimal ionization conditions were achieved in positive ion ESI and APCI using 0.4% formic acid (pH 2.3) and in negative ion ESI and APCI using ammonium acetate buffer (pH 4.0), respectively. MS/MS methods generate information on the molecular weight of individual flavonoids and can often help to distinguish the type and number of sugars attached to aglycone (Table 3.3). However, flavonol glycosides with the same molecular weight (e.g., quercetin 3-glucoside and quercetin 3-galactoside) are not easily resolved by MS methods.

Nonetheless, characteristic fragmentation patterns are associated with the fragmentation of flavonols, and these patterns can often be used to distinguish the aglycone portion of the molecule. For example, a common fragmentation pathway of flavonols such as quercetin, kaempferol, and myricetin is through retro Diels–Alder decomposition, which results in a characteristic and identifying fragment at m/z of 151 in the negative ion mode (Table 3.3). NMR is a powerful tool for the differentiation of isomers, sugar configurations, and substitution patterns on the flavan aromatic ring system. However, NMR has disadvantages such as the extensive sample purification and relatively high amount of analyte required for signal generation. Often, a combination of techniques provides the best compositional information, as seen in a recent study of flavonoid glycosides in the tomato.[37] In this study, LC/MS, ESI(+)/MS/MS, and LC/NMR were used to identify numerous kaempferol glycosides, including kaempferol 3-glucoside, kaempferol 3-rutinoside, kaempferol 3-rutinoside-7-glucoside, and kaempferol 3,7-diglucoside.

GC and thin layer chromatography (TLC) are used less frequently than HPLC for the analysis of flavonols.[79,90,104] To accomplish analysis by GC, flavonols must first be hydrolyzed and converted into trimethylsilyl (TMS) derivatives to increase their volatility and thermal stability. Although this method provides high resolution and low detection limits, it should be noted that TMS derivatives can form with more than one hydroxyl group as they possess different reactivities. This often results in the production of several derivatives, which can complicate quantification. Thus, the

Table 3.3   MS/MS Fragmentation Ions of Flavonoids and Their Metabolites

Compound	M.W.	[M + H]⁺	[M − H]⁻	Fragment Ions
Quercetin	302	303	301	229, 179, 151, 121, 107
Kaempferol	286	287	285	257, 239, 151, 107, 93
Myricetin	318	319	317	151, 137
Isorhamnetin	316	317	315	300
Naringenin	272	273	271	177, 151
Daidzein	254	255	253	223, 208, 133, 91
Daidzin	416	417	415	253
Genistein	270	271	269	241, 225, 201, 197, 133
(+)-Catechin	290	291	289	245, 205
(−)-Epicatechin	290	291	289	245, 205
Cyanidin 3-glucoside	448	449		
Quercetin 3-glucoside	464	465	463	301
Quercetin 3-galactoside	464	465	463	301
Kaempferol 3-glucoside	448	449	447	285
Quercetin 3,7-diglucoside	626	627	625	463, 301
Isorhamnetin 3,7-diglucoside	640	641	639	477, 315
Quercetin 3-rutinoside	610	611	609	301
Quercetin 3-glucuronide	478	479	477	301
Quercetin diglucuronide	654	655	653	477, 301
Quercetin glucoside gluouronide	640	641	639	477, 463
Quercetin glucuronide sulfate	558	559	557	477, 381, 301
Quercetin 3-sulfate	382	383	381	301

Sources: Cited from Mullen, W. et al., *J Chromatogr A*, 1058: 163–168, 2004; Milbury, P. E. et al., *J Agric Food Chem*, 54: 5027–5033, 2006; Franke, A. A. et al., *J Chromatogr B*, 777: 45–59, 2002; Abdel-aal, E. S. M. et al., *J Agric Food Chem*, 54: 4696–4704, 2006.

analysis of flavonols by GC is not generally recommended due to extensive sample cleanup procedures, variable derivatization reactivities, and low reproducibility. Thin layer chromatography still plays a role of the screening of flavonols in plants. Males and Medic-Saric[79] found that the most suitable TLC system for the separation of flavonoids from plant extracts is ethyl acetate:formic acid:water (65:15:20, v/v/v). Pereira et al.[90] developed a high-performance thin layer chromatography method HP/TLC to determine quantitatively flavonoids in *Passiflora* leaves using densitometry, which improved this technique over conventional TLC. HP/TLC has also been employed for the qualitative and quantitative evaluation of flavonoids in *Ginkgo biloba* leaves without cleanup procedures.[58]

Capillary electrophoresis (CE) has also been employed for the analysis of flavonols.[17] In fact, CE methods coupled with electrochemical detection (ECD) are increasingly being employed for the analysis of flavonoids because of the minimal sample volume required, short analysis time, and high separation efficiency.[17] The limit of detection for quercetin and kaempferol by CE/ECD methods are comparable to those obtained by LC/MS. The primary drawback of using CE is low repeatability of retention times as compared with HPLC.

Anthocyanins

Anthocyanins are water soluble pigments responsible for the orange, red, purple, and blue colors of fruits, vegetables, cereals, and flowers. They function to attract pollinators and seed dispersers and also act as photoprotectants, absorbing blue-green light and scavenging free radicals generated during photosynthesis. Anthocyanidins are flavylium (2-phenylchromenylium) cation derivatives. As such, the color of the anthocyanidin is pH dependent. The six primary anthocyanidins widespread in fruits and vegetables include cyanidin, delphinidin, pelargonidin, petunidin, peonidin, and malvidin (Table 3.1). These have in common a hydroxylation of the flavylium ion at the C-3, C-5, and C-7 positions, whereas they differ in the substitution pattern of hydroxyl and/or methoxyl groups on the B-ring. In general, glycosylation occurs with the C-3 hydroxyl position of anthocyanidins, although the C-5 and C-7 hydroxyl groups can also undergo glycosylation. Sugars associated with anthocyanidins include rhamnose, glucose, galactose, and arabinose. In many cases, the sugar residues are acylated by organic acids such as coumaric, caffeic, ferulic, p-hydroxybenzoic, synapic, and malonic acids. Substitution of hydroxyl and methoxyl groups influences the color of anthocyanins. An increase in the number of hydroxyl groups produces deeper blue colors, whereas an increased number of methoxyl groups produces more red color. Anthocyanin stability increases with the number of methoxyl groups in the B-ring and decreases as the number of hydroxyl groups in the B-ring increase. The most stable anthocyanidin is malvidin, followed by peonidin, petunidin, cyanidin and delphinidin. Glycosylation and acylation of the sugars increase anthocyanidin stability and, correspondingly, disaccharides are more stable than their monosaccharide counterparts.

Anthocyanins are generally more stable at an acidic pH. Therefore, anthocyanins are commonly extracted under cold conditions using either acidic methanol or ethanol to avoid degradation[1,51,69] (Table 3.4). In comparison, acetone allows more reproducible extraction and avoids problems with pectins. However, it is limited by the coextraction of proanthocyanins.[39] In general, ethanol is preferable as an extraction solvent, although it can require an additional step for the removal of lipid-soluble substances. SPE using C_{18}, polyamide, HLB (hydrophilic lipophilic balanced stationary phases), or Amberlite has been employed for the purification of anthocyanidins prior to HPLC analysis.[39,51,66,69]

HPLC is the main separation technique for quantification of water-soluble, non-volatile, thermally labile anthocyanins (Table 3.4). The columns most commonly used are reversed-phase C_{18}. The pH of mobile phase is generally kept acidic with either formic, acetic, or trifluoroacetic acid. The order of elution follows the decreasing polarity of the anthocyanidins and is as follows: delphinidin, cyanidin, petunidin, pelargonidin, peonidin, and malvidin. Disaccharide moieties in the C-3 position influence polarity less than the presence of the same two monosaccharides in C-3 and C-5 positions. Anthocyanins absorb visible light at 510–528 nm and UV light at 270–280 nm. DAD is the most common technique used for detection and quantification of anthocyanins, with the quantification occurring around the absorption

Table 3.4 Methodological Overview of Analysis of Anthocyanins from Foods and Biological Samples

Sample	Analytes	Sample Preparation	Column	Mobile Phase	Detection	LOD	Ref.
Baguacu berry	DG, CG, PtG, PG, MG, PgG	Extraction with acidified ethanol, filtration, partitioning, SPE with Amberlite, acid hydrolysis, SPE with C_{18}, derivatization with MSTFA for GC analysis	Cellulose / DB-5 / C-18	EtAc-n-butanol-H_2O-acetic acid-HCl / He / ACN-H_2O-phosphoric acid-acetic acid	TLC (254, 365 nm) / GC/MS / HPLC/MS/MS/ESI(+) or NMR		69
Blackcurrant	CG, CR, DG, DR	Pulverization, partitioning; filtration	Silica and polyacrylamide	Phosphate buffer	CZE/Vis.(520 nm)	CG, CR, DG, 25 mg/L	22
Grape skin, red wine	D, C, Pt, P, M, MG, CG, DG, PG, PtG	Grape skin: extraction with MeOH; Wine: SPE with C_{18}	C-18	MeOH-H_2O-formic acid	HPLC/DAD (530 nm), NMR, HPLC/MS/MS/APCI(−)		66
Mulberry	CG, CR	Extraction with acidified aqueous MeOH, filtration, SPE with polyamide, paper chromatography, alkaline or acid hydrolysis, derivatization for GC analysis	SPB / C-18	He / H_2O-THF-TFA	GC/MS/EI / HPLC/DAD (520 nm)/MS/MS/ESI(+)		51
Radish, red-fleshed potato, juice concentrate	Anthocyanin glycosides	Pulverization, extraction with acetone, filtration, SPE with C_{18}	C-18	ACN-H_2O-phosphoric acid-acetic acid	HPLC/PAD (520 nm), HPLC/MS, or HPLC/MS/MS/ESI(+)		39

(continued on next page)

Table 3.4 (continued) Methodological Overview of Analysis of Anthocyanins from Foods and Biological Samples

Sample	Analytes	Sample Preparation	Column	Mobile Phase	Detection	LOD	Ref.
Red wine	11 Monomeric anthocyanins	Fractionation with gel permeation chromatography	C-18	ACN-H_2O-formic acid	HPLC/DAD (515 nm), HPLC/MS/ESI(+)	0.01 mg/L	44
			Silica	Sodium tetraborate buffer	CZE/DAD		
Standard mixture	CGG, CG, MG, DG, PG, MGG		C-18	ACN-H_2O-formic acid	HPLC/ECD	< 0.3 µM	67
Human plasma and urine	Anthocyanin metabolites	SPE with HLB, centrifugation	Phenyl	ACN-H_2O-formic acid	HPLC/UV-vis (520 nm), HPLC/MS/MS/ESI(+)	0.25 µg/L	21

Notes: LOD, limit of detection; C, cyanidine; D, delphinidine; P, peonidine; M, malvidine; Pt, petunidine; Pg, pelargonidin; CG, cyanidine 3-glucoside; CGG, cyanidine diglucoside; CR, cyanidine 3-rutinoside; DG, delphinidine 3-glucoside; MG, malvidine 3-glucoside; MGG, malvidine diglucoside; PG, peonidine 3-glucoside; PtG, petunidine 3-glucoside; CR, cyaniding 3-rutinoside; DR, delphinidin 3-rutinoiside; MeOH, methanol; ACN, acetonitrile; SPE, solid phase extraction; HLB, hydrophilic lipophilic balanced; THF, tetrahydrofuran; TFA, trifluoroacetic acid; PDA, photodiode array detector; MSTFA, N,O-bis(trimethylsilyl)trifluoroacetamide; GC, gas chromatography; MS, mass spectrometry; HPLC, high-performance liquid chromatography; DAD, diode array detector; CZE, capillary zone electrophoresis; NMR, nuclear magnetic resonance; APCI, atmospheric pressure chemical ionization; ESI, electrospray ionization; ECD, electrochemical detector.

maximum of 520 nm.[1,22,39,51] Glycosylation produces a displacement of the absorption maximum in the visible region of some 10 nm toward lower wavelengths than corresponding aglycone. Phenolic groups attached to the aromatic A- and B-rings can be electrochemically oxidized. Kozminski and Brett[67] used HPLC/ECD to determine anthocyanins using a Ag/AgCl reference electrode. They found that the limit of detection, lower than 0.3 μM, depends on the electrochemical activity of each anthocyanin and also on the potential applied to the electrochemical detector.

In the case of anthocyanins that have no commercially available reference standard, MS and NMR can be used to help elucidate anthocyanidin structure and identify peaks within the HPLC chromatogram. Cooke et al.[21] described the LC/MS/MS method for the identification of anthocyanins in human plasma and urine and suggested the presence of unchanged anthocyanins and anthocyanidin glucuronide metabolites. Kosir et al.[66] identified 13 anthocyanins from wine by the combination of NMR and MS. Anthocyanins are positively charged at acidic pH, are very soluble in water and alcohol, and have relatively low molecular weights. These characteristics permit their easy detection using low voltages because other interfering compounds are usually not ionized. ESI-MS/MS can be used routinely to promote fragmentation of anthocyanidins.

GC coupled to mass spectrometry (GC/MS) and capillary zone electrophoresis (CZE) have also been employed in the analysis of anthocyanins.[51,69] The application of GC/MS after derivatization confirmed only the presence of sugar in anthocyanins.[51,69] Recently, Guadalupe et al.[44] used CE to separate monomeric anthocyanins in an uncoated fused-silica capillary using a borate buffer (pH 9.4) with 10% methanol. However, anthocyanins decompose in the basic condition required for these types of separations. Alternatively, Costa et al.[22] used an acidic running buffer (pH 1.5–2.8) to enhance the detection sensitivity by increasing the number of stable flavylium cations. Acidic running buffers resulted in an increased sensitivity up to 25 $\mu g/mL$, as compared to 4.0 mg/mL obtained using basic running buffers.

Flavan-3-ols and Proanthocyanidins

Flavan-3-ols are mainly composed of (+)-catechin, (–)-epicatechin, (+)-gallocatechin (GC), (–)-epigallocatechin (EGC), (–)-epicatechin-3-gallate (ECG), and (–)-epigallocatechin-3-gallate (EGCG) (Table 3.1). Unlike other flavonoids, flavan-3-ols are often found in condensed forms (dimers, trimers, tetramers, etc.) called proanthocyanidins or condensed tannins. Proanthocyanidins can occur as polymers with degrees of polymerization (DP) above 50 catechin units. Oligomers are primarily linked through the C4-C8 positions or less commonly at the C4-C6 position (B-type interflavan bonds). Examples include procyanidin B_1 (epicatechin-[4β→8]-catechin) and procyanidin B_2 (epicatechin-[4β→8]-epicatechin). A-type proanthocyanidins have a second ether linkage between an A-ring hydroxyl function and the C-2 position of the C-ring. Proanthocyanidins are abundant in numerous foods, including tea, red wine, apples, and cocoa.

Monomeric flavan-3-ols are generally extracted with polar solvents such as water, acetone, methanol, and ethanol with an acid (Table 3.5). Higher molecular weight

EUNMI KOH AND ALYSON E. MITCHELL

Table 3.5 Methodological Overview of Analysis of Flavan-3-ols and Proanthocyanidins from Foods and Biological Samples

Sample	Analytes	Sample Preparation	Column	Mobile Phase	Detection	LOD	Ref.
Anisophyllea dichostyla root bark	C, EC, EGC, ECG, EGCG procyanidin B_1 and B_2, (epi) catechin trimer	Fat removal with hexane, extraction with MeOH, fractionation with silica gel 60	C-18	ACN-H_2O-acetic acid	HPLC/UV/MS/ ESI(−),HPLC/ MS /MS/ ESI(+/−), or NMR		62
Apple	C, EC, EGC, ECG, EGCG	Freeze-drying, pulverization, extraction with MeOH-H_2O	C-18	ACN-phosphate buffer	HPLC/UV (270 nm)/FD (280/310 nm)	C: UV 1.8, FD 0.1 EC: UV 1.2, FD 0.1 µg/g	5
Apple	C, EC, procyanidin B_2	Extraction with aqueous acetone, centrifugation; normal phase: neutralization, SPE with C_{18}; reversed phase: removal of acetone	Silica / C-18	MeOH-DCM-formic acid / MeOH-H_2O-formic acid	HPLC/DAD (280 nm)		112
Ginkgo biloba	C, EC	Pulverization, sonication in MeOH	Silica	Tetraborate-borate buffer	CE/ECD	C 0.17; EC 0.20 mg/L	12
Green tea	C, EC, GC, EGC, GCG, EGCG	Dilution	Silica / C-18	Phosphate-tetraborate-SDS buffer / ACN-H_2O-MeOH-formic acid	HPCE/UV-vis (200 nm) HPLC/DAD (270 nm)	C: LC 0.224, CE 0.0012 EC: LC 0.321, CE 0.0023 mg/L	8

Tea	C, EC, EGC, ECG, EGCG	Extraction with boiling water, filtration	Silica	SDS-phosphate-MeOH buffer	MEKC/UV (200 nm)	C and EC 1.0, EGC 2.0, ECG 3.0, EGCG 6.0 mg/L	6
Tea	C, EC, CG, EGC, EGCG	Extraction with boiling water, followed by aqueous ACN, centrifugation	C-18 Silica	ACN-H_2O-TFA Borate-ACN-phosphate buffer-β cyclodextrin	HPLC/DAD (205 nm) CE/DAD (205 nm)	0.05 mg/L	73
Tea	EGCG, EGC, ECG, EC	Sonication in aqueous EtOH, centrifugation, derivatization	Silica	Ethyl formate-toluene-formic acid-H_2O	HPTLC/UV (366 nm)		96
Human plasma	C	Protein precipitation, centrifugation	C-18	Ammonium phosphate buffer-ACN	HPLC/UV (280 nm) or FD (280/310 nm)	UV, 1 mg/L, FD, 5 µg/L	13
Human and rat serum, plasma and urine	C	Extraction with EtAc, centrifugation, derivatization with BSTFA, enzymatic hydrolysis for conjugates	DB-5	He	GC/MS/SIM	0.01 µg/L	104

Notes: LOD, limit of detection; C, (+)-catechin; EC, (−)-epicatechin; CG, (+)-catechin gallate; ECG, (−)-epicatechin gallate; EGC, (−)-epigallocatechin; GCG, gallocatechingallate; EGCG, (−)-epigallocatechin gallate; MeOH, methanol; EtO-H, ethanol; ACN, acetonitrile; EtAc, ethyl acetate; SPE, solid phase extraction; TFA, trifluoroacetic acid; HPTLC, high-performance thin layer chromatography; MS, mass spectrometry; HPLC, high-performance liquid chromatography; HPCE, high-performance capillary electrophoresis; DAD, diode array detector; FD, fluorescence cetector; CE, capillary electrophoresis; NMR, nuclear magnetic resonance; ESI, electrospray ionization; ECD, electrochemical detector; SDS, sodium dodecyl-sulphate; MEKC, micellar electrokinetic capillary chromatography; BSTFA, bis(trimethylsilyl)trifluoroacetamide; SIM, selection monitoring; DCM, dichlormethane.

oligomers and polymers are more difficult to extract as they form hydrogen-bonds with peptides and proteins. These oligomers generally require a mixture of alcohol, water, and acid (usually 70:29:1 v/v/v) to disrupt hydrogen bonds and facilitate extraction. Arts and Hollman[5] compared the extraction efficiency of three solvents: ethanol, methanol, and acetone. The extraction solvents chosen were 90% methanol for apples and grapes and 70% methanol for beans. The higher proportion of methanol appears to help inactivate polyphenol oxidase—the enzyme responsible for the oxidation and polymerization of catechins during sample preparation. Infusion of samples with hot water is not recommended during extractions, as it can increase the degradation of catechins. Moreover, exposure to high temperatures can cause the inversion of the stereocenter at C-2 of the catechins. Because flavan-3-ols exist as aglycones in most foods, hydrolysis steps are not required. SPE with C_{18} phase is commonly used for the isolation of the flavan-3-ols.

Flavan-3-ols are generally quantified using HPLC and C_{18} columns. The mobile phase used in reversed-phase HPLC methods is generally acetonitrile, methanol, and water with a small amount of an acid to minimize peak tailing. Tetrahydrofuran and dichloromethane are also often used. Typical wavelengths for quantification of flavan-3-ols are 200, 270, or 280 nm. EGC, EGCG, and ECG have little native fluorescence.[5] Thus, one can monitor (+)-catechin and (−)-epicatechin with fluorescence detection and EGC, EGCG, and ECG with UV detection at 270 nm. UV limits of detection of EGCG and ECG (both 0.03 µg/mL) are approximately fourfold higher than (+)-catechin and (−)-epicatechin with fluorescence detection. EGC has the highest limit of detection (LOD, 0.3 µg/mL). In human plasma, fluorescence detection (LOD, 5 ug/L) is 200-fold more sensitive than UV detection (1 mg/L).[13] Additionally, Lee et al.[72] reported lower detection limits using a coulochem electrode array detection (EGC, 1.5 ng/mL; EGCG, 0.5 ng/mL).

There are a few examples of catechins analysis by CE.[8,12,73] For the separation of catechins in green tea extract, Bonoli et al.[8] demonstrated that high-performance capillary electrophoresis (HPCE) has higher sensitivity (20–100 times lower LOD) and shorter analysis times than HPLC (12 vs. 40 minutes). However, HPLC methods display better repeatability for the quantification of catechins. In contrast, Lee and Ong[73] reported that CE was 10-fold less sensitive than HPLC, although it was three times faster. The use of a borate–phosphate–SDS buffer system resulted in better resolution of catechins in CE.[71] In general, consistency and reproducibility are harder to achieve using CE methods. Catechins have also been analyzed using HP/TLC on cellulose[111] or silica plates.[96] Although LC/MS/MS methods are robust and have been applied to characterize the structures of catechins,[62,76] these methods are limited because they cannot distinguish between stereoisomers such as (+)-catechin and (−)-epicatechin, which have identical mass fragmentation patterns and ions (Table 3.3).

Isoflavones

Unlike other flavonoids, isoflavones are flavonoids with the B-ring attached at the C-3 position of the C-ring (Table 3.1). Isoflavones are present predominantly in soy foods and are found as O-glycosidic conjugates and as acetylated and malo-nylated O-glycosidic conjugates including 6"-O-malonyl-β-glycoside, 6"-O-acetyl-β-glycoside, and β-glycoside.[23,42,87,92,98] Glycosylation occurs mainly at the C-7 position, with the exception of puerarin, (8-C-glucosyldaidzein) found in kudzu.[92] In raw soybeans, malonyl forms predominate. In comparison, fermented foods or processed soy foods contain relatively high levels of the aglycones and β-glycosides as glycosidic bonds, and ester bonds in malonyl or acetyl forms are hydrolyzed by microbial enzymes (e.g., β-glucosidase) and heat processing.[23,65] Isoflavone aglycones have limited solubility in both water and organic solvents. In contrast, the glycosidic conjugates are highly water soluble. Because malonyl and acetyl glycosidic forms are susceptible to heat and readily convert into β-glycosides, extractions at elevated tem-peratures may cause changes in the composition of isoflavones measured in foods.

To carry out quantitative measurement of isoflavones using chromatographic methods, internal standards are commonly used to correct for losses during extrac-tion and sample preparation. The most common internal standards include deuterated (^{2}H)- or carbon-13 (^{13}C)-labeled isoflavones and compounds with similar chemical properties that are not naturally present in the sample—for example, fluorescein, flavone, formononetin, apigenin, and biochanin A (Table 3.6). Soxhlet extraction or ultrasonication with organic solvents is the prevailing technique for the extraction of isoflavones from food matrices. The solvents commonly used for isoflavone extrac-tion are methanol, ethanol, acetone, or acetonitrile. Murphy et al.[87] attempted to determine the optimum extraction solvent for various isoflavone forms present in soy foods. Acetonitrile was superior to other solvents in extracting 12 isoflavone com-pounds.[42,87] Nevertheless, it was suggested that each food must be initially evaluated to determine the optimum extraction protocol such as the extraction time and the ratio of acetonitrile to water. Recently, supercritical fluid extraction (SFE) has been applied as an alternative to conventional approaches.[63] SFE uses relatively mild sepa-ration conditions that minimize the degradation of intact isoflavones in foods or their metabolites in biological samples. Furthermore, detection limits were significantly improved with SFE as compared to conventional extraction methods.

Soy isoflavones undergo extensive metabolism in animals after consumption. Examination of biological samples (e.g., plasma, serum, and urine) after soy con-sumption demonstrates that soy isoflavones are metabolized to β-glucuronides and sulfate esters. Enzymatic hydrolysis of soy isoflavone metabolites is a common procedure for determining the total isoflavone in biological fluids. To accomplish this, the sample is treated with a mixture of β-glucuronidase and sulfatase prior to analysis of the isoflavones. To confirm the efficiency of enzymatic hydrolysis, phenolphthalein glucuronide and methylumbelliferone glucuronide can be used as internal standards.[24] After enzymatic hydrolysis, sample preparation procedures for aglycones include solvent extraction using ethyl ether, protein precipitation with acetonitrile, and liquid–liquid partitioning with hexane to remove lipids. In addition, sugars can be removed using SPE with C_{18} cartridges. This step can also be used to concentrate the samples prior to HPLC analysis.

The use of HPLC coupled with ECD, DAD, and/or MS detection is typical for the determination of isoflavones. Separation by HPLC has been used extensively

Table 3.6 Methodological Overview of Isoflavone Analysis from Foods and Biological Samples

Sample	Analytes	Sample Preparation	Column (i.s.)	Mobile Phase	Detection	LOD	Ref.
Puerariae radix root	D, BCA, G, daidzin, puerarin	Ultrasonication in MeOH, filtration	Silica	Borax-NaOH buffer	CE/UV (200 nm)	1.2–1.8 mg/L	113
Red clover	D, G, FORM, ononin, BCA, sissotrin, their glycosides	Ultrasonication in MeOH-H_2O-Tris buffer	C-18	MeOH-ammonium formate	HPLC/UV (265 nm), FD (250/418 nm) or MS/APCI(−)	UV 20–90 mg/L	98
Red clover, soy bits	D, G, GLY, ononin, sissotrin	Ultrasonication, SFE	C-18 (flavone)	ACN-H_2O-acetic acid	HPLC/DAD/ MS/ ESI(−)/SIM	0.2–3.6 fmol	63
Soy-based milk formula	D, G, FORM, BCA	Reflux with 80% ethanol, centrifugation, partitioning Conjugates: enzymatic hydrolysis, SPE with C_{18}	C-18	MeOH-ammonium acetate	HPLC/UV (260 nm), ECD or MS	UV 5 ng, ED 10–15 pg	103
Soy foods	D, G	Extraction with 80% MeOH, centrifugation, partitioning	C-8 (fluorescein)	ACN-H_2O-TFA	HPLC/UV (262 nm)		23
Soy protein and foods, nutritional supplements	D, G, GLY, their conjugates	Extraction with aqueous ACN, centrifugation	C-18 (apigenin)	ACN-H_2O-acetic acid	HPLC/UV (260 nm)/MS^n/ ESI(+)	0.4–1.0 µg/L	42

Human plasma	D, DHD, G, ODMA	Acidification, enzymatic hydrolysis, extraction with C_{18} SPE or diethyl ether, partitioning	C-8 (Phenolphthalein glucuronide, 4-methylumbelliferone glucuronide, BCA)	$ACN-H_2O$-ammonium acetate	HPLC/MS/MS/APCI($-$)	24
Human urine	D, G, equol, ODMA	Acidification, extraction with C_{18} SPE, anion exchangers (DEAE and QAE), enzymatic hydrolysis, silylation	BP-1 (deuterated isoflavones)	He	GC/MS/EI	2
Human urine and blood	D, DHD, G, DHG, ODMA	Centrifugation, enzymatic hydrolysis, extraction with ethyl ether	C-18 (formononetin)	MeOH-ACN-H_2O-acetic acid	HPLC/DAD/MS/MS/ESI($-$)	35
Urine	D, G	Extraction with SPME fiber or C-18 SPE	C-18	MeOH-H_2O	HPLC/MS/MS/ESI($+$)/SIM	99

Notes: LOD, limit of detection; i.s., internal standard; D, daidzein; G, genistein; FORM, formononetin; BCA, biochanin A; GIY, glycitein; DHD, dihydrodaidzein; DHG, dihydrogenistein; ODMA, O-desmethylangolensin; MeOH, methanol: ACN, acetonitrile; SPE, solid phase extraction; SPME, solid phase microextraction; SFE, supercritical fluid extraction; ; TFA, trifluoroacetic acid; GC, gas chromatography; MS, mass spectrometry; HPLC, high-performance liquid chromatography; DAD, diode array detector; FD, fluorescence detector; ESI, electrospray ionization; NMR, nuclear magnetic resonance; APCI, atmospheric pressure chemical ionization; CE, capillary electrophoresis; ECD, electrochemical detector; DEAE, diethyl-aminoethyl; QAE, quarternary amino ethyl; EI, electron impact; SIM, select ion monitoring.

with UV and/or fluorescence detection. The weakness of these detection methods is their nonspecificity, leading to the possibility of sample matrix interference. In general, the mobile phases employed with reversed-phase HPLC columns are acetonitrile and/or methanol in combination with water containing a small amount of an acid (0.1–1% acetic, formic, or trifluoroacetic acid). The most often used columns are packed with reversed-phase C_{18} column material, but sometimes C_8 columns are employed. Isoflavones absorb UV light with a maximum wavelength in the range of 250 to 270 nm. Both isocratic and gradient elution methods have been applied to isoflavone separations. Setchell et al.[103] described a simple isocratic reversed-phase method using methanol and 0.1 M ammonium acetate (pH 4.6) as the mobile phase. Isoflavones that are naturally fluorescent are limited to daidzein and formononetin. Therefore, postcolumn derivatization with aluminum is required to detect nonfluorescent genistein and biochanin A by fluorescence detection.

Fluorescence detection provides better selectivity and sensitivity as compared with UV detection. In addition, isoflavones containing a phenol group can be determined by ECD, increasing sensitivity for most isoflavones by a factor of two to six compared to UV detection. However, baseline instability, caused by electro-oxidation of impurities present in the mobile phase, can be a problem. LC/MS/MS is very useful for the characterization of isoflavones, especially for clinical studies of isoflavone metabolites in biological fluids. ESI-LC/MS/MS in the negative mode with an ammonium acetate buffer as the mobile phase modifier provides the best sensitivity.[95] Waridel et al.[114] demonstrated that the loss of a 120-Da fragment is indicative of C-glycosidic isoflavones. In studies comparing APCI and ESI ionization techniques, Prasain et al.[93] reported that the C-glycosidic isoflavone, puerarin, isolated from kudzu supplements was ionized more efficiently in the negative ion mode, with APCI generally giving better ionization than ESI. By selecting unique daughter ions for each isoflavone, multiple reaction ion monitoring (MRM) can be developed as a highly sensitive, quantitative method of analysis. Setchell et al.[103] compared the sensitivities of three kinds of detectors, including HPLC/UV, ECD, or LC/MS/MS employing select ion monitoring (SIM). The detection limits of genistein and daidzein were 5 ng and 10–15 pg for UV and ECD, respectively. MS/MS using SIM resulted in a 100-fold improvement in the sensitivity over UV detection.

Dietary isoflavones contain at least one hydroxyl group in their structure, which makes it difficult for their analysis by GC/MS without derivatization. Electron impact GC/MS has been used for the analysis of isoflavones. However, prior to analysis, TMS ether derivatives were necessary to increase the volatility and thermal stability of the isoflavones.[2] Additionally, a cleanup procedure is usually employed to remove coextracted compounds. Wang et al.[113] separated five isoflavone compounds in *Puerariae radix* within 6 minutes using HPCE in a 20-mM borax–NaOH (pH 10.1) buffer.

Flavanones

Flavanones are predominantly found in citrus fruits such as oranges, grapefruit, and lemons. They are usually present as mono- and diglycosides (Table 3.1).

Flavanone glycosides hesperidin and naringin are responsible for the bitterness in oranges and grapefruit, respectively.

Methanol, acetone, and acetonitrile have been used as solvents for extraction of flavanones in citrus fruits (Table 3.7). Strong alkali solvents may convert flavanones to their chalcone derivatives, which can lead to an underestimation of the contents of flavanones in a sample. The most common HPLC column used to monitor flavanones is the reversed-phase C_{18} column. β-cyclodextrin-bonded columns have also been used, as they make it possible to separate flavanone glycoside diastereomers in *Citrus* extracts.[68] Several liquid chromatographic methods employing UV detection for measuring flavanones have been reported.[10,11,30,68,110] Flavanones and their glycosides are generally detected at 280 nm. The detection limit of eight flavanone compounds by HPLC with UV ranged from 7 to 18 mg/L.[11] HPLC coupled with a conductivity detector demonstrated about 10-fold lower detection limits than HPLC with UV detection for hesperetin and naringenin.[7] CE coupled to ECD has demonstrated even lower detection limits of 30 µg/L for hesperetin.[18] Detection limits of 0.5–1.0 µg/L for naringin and hesperidin in the biological fluids were obtained by LC/MS/MS, demonstrating the usefulness of this method for the measurement of flavanones at lower levels in biological fluids.[38,75]

Carotenoids

Carotenoids are naturally occurring tetraterpenes present in plants, algae, yeasts, and molds (Figure 3.2). These hydrocarbon or xanthophyll compounds are lipid soluble and responsible for many of the yellow and red colors in plants such as the red color of tomato, which is produced by the carotenoid lycopene. Carotenoids are present in free and esterified forms and can have various fatty acids attached to them. The predominant geometric isomer of carotenoids from plant sources is the more thermodynamically stable all-*trans* form. For example, in tomatoes the all-*trans*-lycopene accounts for 79–91% of total lycopene. However, various *cis*-isomers are present in the processed foods as well as human serum and tissues. For example, *cis*-isomers accounted for 79–88% of total lycopene in benign or malignant prostate tissues.[19] These pigments can be extracted with nonpolar solvents such as hexane, dichloromethane, methyl *tert*-butyl ether (MTBE), and ethyl ether (Table 3.8). If the samples are fresh and contain water, polar solvents including acetone, methanol, tetrahydrofuran, or ethyl acetate are added to improve the extraction efficiency of carotenoids. To date, no solvent has proven ideal for the extraction of all carotenoids. Polar solvents are good for the extraction of xanthophylls, whereas the more nonpolar solvents are appropriate for the extraction of hydrocarbon carotenes. The general recommendation is to use a nonpolar solvent containing a low proportion of polar solvent to complete the extraction of carotenoids from foods.[74,101]

Exposure of carotenoids, especially lycopene, to heat and light during cooking or processing may result in *cis-trans* isomerization. Therefore, the extraction should be carried out quickly, avoiding unnecessary exposure to light, oxygen, heat, and pro-oxidant metals such as iron and copper. Furthermore, to help prevent carotenoid losses during extraction procedures, the addition of antioxidants such as

Table 3.7   Methodological Overview of Flavanone Analysis from Foods and Biological Samples

Sample	Analytes	Sample Preparation	Column	Mobile Phase	Detection	LOD	Ref.
Buchu leaves	Diosmin, hesperidin	Reflux with MeOH, filtration	C-18	MeOH-H_2O	HPLC/UV (345 nm)	5 mg/L	30
Citrus juice	Naringin, prunin, narirutin, (neo) hesperidin	SPE with polyamide	β-Cyclodextrin	MeOH-acetic acid-H_2O	HPLC/DAD (280 nm)		68
Citrus juice	Narirutin, (neo) eriocitrin (neo) hesperidin, naringin, didymin	Freeze-dried, extracted with ether or hexane, followed by EtAc, MeOH or ACN	C-18	MeOH-H_2O-acetic acid	HPLC/DAD (280 nm)	7–18 mg/L	11
Flos chrysanthemum	Hesperetin	Pulverization, ultrasonication in aqueous EtOH, centrifugation	Silica	Tetraborate-borate buffer	CE/ECD	30 μg/L	18
Herbs	Eriodictyol, hesperetin, naringenin	Freeze-dried, pulverization, extraction with aqueous MeOH	C-18	H_2O-MeOH-formic acid	HPLC/DAD/ MS^n/APCI(−)		59
Orange, grapefruit, lemon	Naringenin, hesperetin	Peeling, separation for juice and albedo, air-dried, derivatization with TMS-(oxime)ether, acid hydrolysis for glycosides	ID-BPX5	He	GC/MS/ ion trap detector		36

Matrix	Compounds	Sample preparation	Column	Mobile phase	Method/detection	LOD	Ref.
Orange juice, grape juice	Naringin, hesperidin, narirutin	Extraction with MeOH, centrifugation, glass fiber filtration	C-18	H_2O-TFA, 2-propanol-formic acid-H_2O	HPLC/ UV-vis. (283 nm)		10
Oregano	Eriodictyol, naringenin	Dried, pulverization, soxhlet in acetone	C-18	ACN-H_2O-formic acid	HPLC/UV (280 nm)/SPE/ NMR or LC/ MS/MS/ESI(−)		31
Phytomedicine	Hesperetin, naringenin	Extracted with ACN	Polyimide-silica	Background electrolyte buffer	CE/UV (214 nm) CE/CD	CD, 0.17, 0.15; UV, 1.02, 1.2C mg/L	7
Standard mixture	Naringenin		Silica	EtAc-tuolene-cyclohexane-formic acid-n-hexane-acetic acid	TLC/UV (254, 366 nm)		81
Human blood, plasma	Naringenin, hesperetin	Sonication in acidic MeOH, enzymatic hydrolysis, extraction with EtAc, centrifugation	C-18	ACN-H_2O-formic acid	HPLC/DAD (290 nm)/MS/ MS/ESI(−)	Naringenin 0.5 µg/L, hesperetin 1.0 µg/L	38
Rat serum	Naringin, (neo)hesperidin	SPE with HLB copolymer	C-18	ACN-H_2O	HPLC/MS/MS/ APCI(−)	0.7 µg/L	75

Notes: LOD, limit of detection; MeOH, methanol; EtOH, ethanol; ACN, acetonitrile; EtAC, ethyl acetate; SPE, solid phase extraction; HLB (hydrophilic lipophilic balanced); TFA, trifluoroacetic acid; GC, gas chromatography; TMS, trimethylsilyl; MS, mass spectrometry; HPLC, high-performance liquid chromatography; DAD, diode array detector; NMR, nuclear magnetic resonance; ESI, electrospray ionization; APCI, atmospheric pressure chemical ionization; CE, capillary electrophoresis; ECD, electrochemical detector; CD, conductivity detector; TLC, thin layer chromatography; PDA, photodiode array detector.

Table 3.8 Methodological Overview of Carotenoid Analysis from Foods and Biological Samples

Sample	Analytes	Sample Preparation	Column	Mobile Phase	Detection	LOD	Ref.
Crude standard	Astaxanthin		Silica	Hexane-acetone-THF	HPLC/DAD/MS/ESI(+)/NMR		94
Marigold flower extract	Zeaxanthin, lutein, lutein ester, their isomers	Saponification with KOH, neutralization, extraction with ethyl ether	Silica and β-cyclobond C-30	n-Hexane-ethyl acetate MeOH-MTBE	HPLC/UV-vis (450 nm) MS/ESI(+)		46
Orange juice	9 carotenoids	Centrifugation, saponification with KOH, extraction with DCM	C-18	ACN-MeOH-DCM-H_2O	HPLC/UV-vis (454 nm)	0.22 μmol for β-carotene	82
Plant extract	12 carotenoids	Saponification, extraction with diethyl ether, SPE with silica	C-18	Petroleum-MeOH-ACN	TLC		57
Pumpkin, tunicate, oyster	Epoxy carotenoids	Extraction with acetone, partitioning, fractioned with silica, purified with HPLC using C_{18}		Chloroform-ACN	MS/MS/FAB(+)		80
Standard mixture	β-carotene, lycopene, canthaxanthin, lutein, zeaxanthin		C-30	Acetone-H_2O-$AgClO_4$	HPLC/UV-vis (450 nm)/MS/MS/ESI(+)	0.5, 0.3 pmol for canthaxanthin and β-carotene	97
Tomato	Lycopene isomers, β-carotene	SFE	C-30	MeOH-H_2O-MTBE	HPLC/PAD (285, 347, 450 nm)		40

Sample	Analytes	Extraction	Column	Mobile phase	Detection	LOD	Ref.
Tomato, human prostate	Lycopene isomers, α/β-carotene	Tomato: extraction with acetone-hexane; Prostate: protein precipitation, extraction with acetone-hexane	C-30	MeOH-MTBE-ammonium acetate	HPLC/ECD	50 fmol for lycopene	34
Vegetable juice	β-carotene isomers, astaxanthin, zeaxanthin, canthaxanthin, echinenone	Extraction with MTBE, photo isomerization	C-30	MeOH-MTBE	HPLC/DAD (450 nm)/MS/APCI(+)	1 pmol for β-carotene	70
Human plasma	Lycopene isomers, α/β/γ-carotene	Extraction with hexane, centrifugation, saponification with KOH	C-18/C-30	ACN-MTBE	HPLC/MS/MS/APCI(+/−)	11.2 fmol for lycopene	32
Human serum	Lycopene, lutein, β-carotene, β-crytoxanthin, zeaxanthin	Protein precipitation, extraction with n-hexane	C-30	MeOH-ACN-THF-BHT	HPLC/DAD (450 nm)	<0.06 μmol	45
Human serum, prostate	Lycopene isomers, α/β-carotene	Saponification with KOH, extraction with hexane, centrifugation	C-30	MeOH-MTBE	HPLC/PDA (450 nm)/MS/APCI(+)	0.93 pmol for lycopene	109

Notes: LOD, limit of detection; MeOH, methanol; EtOH, ethanol; ACN, acetonitrile; MTBE, methyl tert-butyl ether; DCM, dichloromethane; THF, tetrahydrofuran; KOH, potassium hydroxide; SFE, supercritical fluid extraction; HPLC, high-performance liquid chromatography; DAD, diode array detector; PDA, photodiode array detector; FD, fluorescence detector; ECD, electrochemical detector; ESI, electrospray ionization; APCI, atmosphere pressure chemical ionization; TLC, thin layer chromatography; FAB, fast atom bombardment; NMR, nuclear magnetic resonance; BHT, butylated hydroxytoluene; SPE, solid phase extraction.

butylhydroxytoluene (BHT) and pyrogallol can be used.[19,32,82,109] Additionally, extraction efficiencies can be improved by carrying out procedures in dim light.[45] SPE on silica has been used to fractionate carotenoids prior to HPLC analysis.[80] SFE offers advantages such as rapidity, controlled solvent strength, and low toxicity. For these reasons, SFE using CO_2 has been used for the isolation of carotenoids from various plants. However, there is a limitation of quantitative extraction of polar compounds from solid matrices. Careri et al.[14] optimized the extraction of carotenoids from *Spirulina pacifica* algae by evaluating the effects of four parameters: temperature, pressure, time, and percentage of ethanol added as a modifier. The addition of a modifier resulted in an increase of extraction yield by changing the polarity of the extraction fluid. In another study, Gomez-Prieto et al.[40] used SFE with no additional modifiers to extract all-*trans*-lycopene from tomatoes. This helped to minimize the isomerization and oxidation of lycopene, leading to improved isolation efficiency of the more stable all-*trans* form of lycopene. The extract contained 88% all-*trans*-lycopene and 12% *cis*-lycopene.

Saponification is often used to extract xanthophylls as well as remove chlorophylls and lipids from samples prior to analysis, as these compounds can interfere with the chromatographic detection. Although saponification with methanol and potassium hydroxide is routinely used to facilitate carotenoid extraction, numerous studies indicate that saponification can also result in losses of carotenoids. For example, Khachik et al.[60] demonstrated that saponification actually caused the loss of total carotenoids in samples. Alternatively, enzymatic saponification using lipase can be used to help prevent the loss and isomerization of some carotenoids. Fang et al.[32] suggested that saponification of plasma samples should be avoided to prevent unnecessary lycopene degradation.

HPLC is commonly used to separate and quantify carotenoids using C_{18} and, more efficiently, on C_{30} stationary phases, which led to superior separations and improved peak shape.[32,40,46] An isocratic reversed-phase HPLC method for routine analysis of carotenoids was developed using the mobile phase composed of either methanol:acetonitrile:methylene chloride:water (50:30:15:5 v/v/v/v)[82] or methanol:acetonitrile:tetrahydrofuran (75:20:5 v/v/v).[45] This method was achieved within 30 minutes, whereas gradient methods for the separation of carotenoids can be more than 60 minutes. Normal-phase HPLC has also been used for carotenoid analyses using β-cyclobond[46] and silica stationary phases.[94] The reversed-phase methods employing C_{18} and C_{30} stationary phases achieved better separation of individual isomers. The *cis*-isomers of lycopene, lutein, and β-carotene are often identified by comparing their spectral characteristic Q ratios and/or the relative retention times of the individual isomers obtained from iodine/heat-isomerized lycopene solutions.[16,34,46,70,74,101] However, these methods alone cannot be used for the identification of numerous carotenoids isomers that co-elute (e.g., 13-*cis* lycopene and 15-*cis* lycopene). In the case of compounds whose standards are not available, additional techniques such as MS and NMR are required for complete structural elucidation and validation.

Carotenoids are typically detected at the wavelength of maximum absorption of 450–470 nm. The detection and quantification of carotenoids at very low levels, especially in biological samples, require the development of improved methodology to increase sensitivity and selectivity. ECD has been successfully applied to significantly increase sensitivity for β-carotene, α-carotene, lutein, and zeaxanthin.[33] Since biological samples usually contain a number of electrochemically active components beyond the carotenoids of interest, interferences may occur with single-channel ECD, which can decrease sensitivity. Therefore, determination of geometric isomers of carotenoids such as lycopene in biological fluids and tissues requires more selective techniques than single-channel HPLC/ECD. For example, Ferruzzi et al.[34] applied both four-channel isocratic and eight-channel gradient ECD methods using different proportions of methanol, MTBE, water, and 1 M ammonium acetate buffer for carotenoid separations in human tissues. The gradient method simultaneously separated both carotenes and 12 lycopene isomers in human cervical tissue with 10- to 100-fold improved detection limits as compared to UV-Vis absorbance detection methods.

To increase the sensitivity and selectivity of carotenoid analysis, LC/MS methods have been developed using continuous-flow fast atom bombardment,[15,80] ESI,[97] and APCI.[32,70,109] Because carotenoids are relatively nonpolar compounds that often lack a site for protonation, their ionization for mass spectrometric detection is not simple. APCI ionization methods are preferred, as these resulted in improved ionization and sensitivity for the quantitative analysis of lycopene isomers in human serum and prostate tissue.[109] Diagnostic fragmentation ions demonstrate good linearity and reproducibility for lycopene.[109] The limits of detection of carotenoids with APCI-LC/MS/MS methods are substantially improved in the picomole and even femtomole levels.[32,70,109] Fang et al.[32] suggested that lycopene should be injected within 30 minutes after extraction and that its half-life is ~16 hours in a temperature-controlled autosampler at 4°C. Hydrocarbon carotenoids (e.g., lycopene and carotenes) lack a site for protonation or proton removal and therefore are difficult to analyze by ESI/MS. Rentel et al.[97] added Ag^+ to the chromatographic eluent to enhance the ionization of carotenoids in the ESI/MS and achieved the detection limit of 0.5 and 0.3 pmol for canthaxanthin and β-carotene, respectively. However, silver salts produce clusters in the lower mass range and, therefore, mass spectral scans are only effective above 400 m/z, although this can depend upon the ratio of analytes to silver ions as well as the solvent composition. Khachik et al.[61] recently isolated and identified (13Z,13'Z,3R,3'R,6'R)-lutein in kale and human plasma by comparison of the HPLC retention times (as determined by UV-visible), MS, and NMR.

TLC methods were employed to isolate 12 carotenoid compounds by Isaksen and Francis.[57] To date, TLC is often used as the first identification step for carotenoids. GC is almost never applied for carotenoid analysis due to carotenoids' thermal instability.

CONCLUSIONS

The characterization and quantification of the complement of flavonoids and carotenoids in foods and biological samples will be of continued interest, especially with respect to determining their contribution to and role in human health and disease prevention. Because these compounds often exist at trace levels in complex natural matrices and various biological samples, the development of selective and sensitive analytical methods is still required. Moreover, improved understanding and development of mild sample preparation conditions will be necessary in order to evaluate the natural distribution of flavonoids, their glycosides, and carotenoid isomers in foods and biological tissues. HPLC, in conjunction with DAD or UV-visible detectors, offers sufficient quantitative results for both groups of phytochemicals. However, the optimization of the mobile and stationary phase combinations can still be improved.

Further developments in soft ionization tandem MS and NMR detection methods will lead to improvements of our understanding of the endogenous structures of these compounds and will help identify physiological pathways relating to the metabolism of these compounds.

REFERENCES

1. Abdel-aal, ESM, Young JC and Rabalski I, Anthocyanin composition in black, blue, pink, purple, and red cereal grains. *J Agric Food Chem* 54: 4696–4704 (2006).
2. Adlercreutz H, Wildt J, Kinzel J, Attalla H, Wahala K, Makela T, Hase T and Fotsis T, Lignan and isoflavonoid conjugates in human urine. *J Steroid Biochem Molec Biol* 52: 97–103 (1995).
3. Alaniya MD, Kinetics of the alkaline hydrolysis of flavonoid glycosides. *Chem Nat Compounds* 13: 536–539 (1978).
4. Andrade FDP, Santos LC, Datchler M, Albert K and Vilegas W, Use of online liquid chromatography–nuclear magnetic resonance spectroscopy for the rapid investigation of flavonoids from *Sorocea bomplandii*. *J Chromatogr A* 953: 287–291 (2002).
5. Arts ICW and Hollman PCH, Optimization of a quantitative method for the determination of catechins in fruits and legumes. *J Agric Food Chem* 46: 5156–5162 (1998).
6. Aucamp JP, Hara Y and Apostolides Z, Simultaneous analysis of tea catechins, caffeine, gallic acid, theanine and ascorbic acid by micellar electrokinetic capillary chromatography. *J Chromatogr A* 876: 235–242 (2000).
7. Bachmann S, Huck CW, Bakry R and Bonn GK, Analysis of flavonoids by CE using capacitively coupled contactless conductivity detection. *Electrophoresis* 28: 799–805 (2007).
8. Bonoli M, Pelillo M, Toschi TG and Lercker G, Analysis of green tea catechins: Comparative study between HPLC and HPCE. *Food Chem* 81: 631–638 (2003).
9. Brandt S, Pek Z, Barna E, Lugasi A and Helyes L, Lycopene content and color of ripening tomatoes as affected by environmental conditions. *J Sci Food Agric* 86: 568–572 (2006).
10. Bronner WE and Beecher GR, Extraction and measurement of prominent flavonoids in orange and grapefruit juice concentrates. *J Chromatogr A* 705: 247–256 (1995).
11. Calabro ML, Galtieri V, Cutroneo P, Tommasini S, Ficarra P and Ficarra R, Study of the extraction procedure by experimental design and validation of a LC method for determination of flavonoids in *Citrus bergamia* juice. *J Pharm Biomed Anal* 35: 349–363 (2004).
12. Cao Y, Chu Q, Fang Y and Ye J, Analysis of flavonoids in *Ginkgo biloba* L. and its phytopharmaceuticals by capillary electrophoresis with electrochemical detection. *Anal Bioanal Chem* 374: 294–299 (2002).
13. Carando S, Teissedre PL and Cabanis JC, Comparison of (+)-catechin determination in human plasma by high-performance liquid chromatography with two types of detection: Fluorescence and ultraviolet. *J Chromatogr B* 707: 195–201 (1998).

14. Careri M, Furlattini L, Mangia A, Musci M, Anklam E, Theobald A and von Holst C, Supercritical fluid extraction for liquid chromatographic determination of carotenoids in *Spirulina pacifica* algae: A chemometric approach. *J Chromatogr A* 912: 61–71 (2001).

15. Caccamese S and Garozzo D, Odd-electron molecular ion and loss of toluene in fast atom bombardment mass spectra of some carotenoids. *Org Mass Spectrom* 25: 137–140 (1990).

16. Chen BH, Peng HY and Chen HE, Changes of carotenoids, color, and vitamin A contents during processing of carrot juice. *J Agric Food Chem* 43: 1912–1918 (1995).

17. Chen G, Zhang H and Ye J, Determination of rutin and quercetin in plants by capillary electrophoresis with electrochemical detection. *Anal Chim Acta* 423: 69–76 (2000).

18. Chu Q, Fu L, Guan Y and Ye J, Determination and differentiation of *Flos chrysanthemum* based on characteristic electrochemical profiles by capillary electrophoresis with electrochemical detection. *J Agric Food Chem* 52: 7828–7833 (2004).

19. Clinton SK, Emenhiser C, Schwartz SJ, Bostwick DG, Williams AW, Moore BJ and Erdman JW, Jr, *Cis-trans* lycopene isomers, carotenoids, and retinol in the human prostate. *Cancer Epidemiol Biomarkers Prev* 5: 823–833 (1996).

20. Commenges D, Scotet V, Renaud S, Jacqmin-Gadda H, Barberger-Gateau P and Dartigues JF, Intake of flavonoids and risk of dementia. *Eur J Epidemiol* 16: 357–363 (2000).

21. Cooke DN, Thomasset S, Boocock DJ, Schwarz M, Winterhalter P, Steward WP, Gescher AJ and Marczylo TH, Development of analyses by high-performance liquid chromatography and liquid chromatography/tandem mass spectrometry of bilberry (*Vaccinium myrtilus*) anthocyanins in human plasma and urine. *J Agric Food Chem* 54: 7009–7013 (2006).

22. da Costa CT, Nelson BC, Margolis SA and Horton D, Separation of blackcurrant anthocyanins by capillary zone electrophoresis. *J Chromatogr A* 799: 321–327 (1998).

23. Coward L, Barnes NC, Setchell KDR and Barnes S, Genistein, daidzein, and their β-glycoside conjugates: Antitumor isoflavones in soybean foods from American and Asian diets. *J Agric Food Chem* 41: 1961–1967 (1993).

24. Coward L, Kirk M, Albin N and Barnes S, Analysis of plasma isoflavones by reversed-phase HPLC-multiple reaction ion monitoring–mass spectrometry. *Clin Chim Acta* 247: 121–142 (1996).

25. Crozier A, Lean MEJ, McDonald MS and Black C, Quantitative analysis of the flavonoid content of commercial tomatoes, onions, lettuce, and celery. *J Agric Food Chem* 45: 590–595 (1997).

26. Delgado-Vargas F, Jimenez AR and Paredes-Lopez O, Natural pigments: Carotenoids, anthocyanins, and betalains—Characteristics, biosynthesis, processing, and stability. *Crit Rev Food Sci Nutr* 40: 173–289 (2000).

27. Dixon R and Paiva N, Stress-induced phenylpropanoid metabolism. *Plant Cell* 7: 1085–1097 (1995).

28. Dubber MJ, Sewram V, Mshicileli N, Shephard GS and Kanfer I, The simultaneous determination of selected flavonols glycosides and aglycones in *Ginkgo biloba* oral dosage forms by high-performance liquid chromatography–electrospray ionization–mass spectrometry. *J Pharm Biomed Anal* 37: 723–731 (2005).

29. Duthie G and Crozier A, Plant-derived phenolic antioxidants. *Curr Opin Lipidol* 11: 43–47 (2000).

30. El-Shafae AM and El-Domiaty MM, Improved LC methods for the determination of diosmin and/or hesperidin in plant extracts and pharmaceutical formulations. *J Pharm Biomed Anal* 26: 539–545 (2001).

31. Exarchou V, Godejohann M, van Beek TA, Gerothanassis IP and Vervoort J, LC–UV–solid phase extraction–NMR–MS combined with a cryogenic flow probe and its application to the identification of compounds present in Greek oregano. *Anal Chem* 75: 6288–6294 (2003).
32. Fang L, Pajkovic N, Wang Y, Gu C and van Breemen RB, Quantitative analysis of lycopene isomers in human plasma using high-performance liquid chromatography–tandem mass spectrometry. *Anal Chem* 75: 812–817 (2003).
33. Ferruzzi MG, Sander LC, Rock CL and Schwartz SJ, Carotenoid determination in biological microsamples using liquid chromatography with a coulometric electrochemical array detector. *Anal Chem* 74: 256–281 (1998).
34. Ferruzzi MG, Nguyen ML, Sander LC, Rock CL and Schwartz SJ, Analysis of lycopene geometrical isomers in biological microsamples by liquid chromatography with coulometric array detection. *J Chromatogr B* 760: 289–299 (2001).
35. Franke AA, Custer LJ, Wilkens LR, Marchand LL, Nomura AMY, Goodman MT and Kolonel LN, Liquid chromatographic–photodiode array mass spectrometric analysis of dietary phytoestrogens from human urine and blood. *J Chromatogr B* 777: 45–59 (2002).
36. Fuzfai Z and Molnar-Perl I, Gas chromatographic–mass spectrometric fragmentation study of flavonoids as their trimethylsilyl derivatives: Analysis of flavonoids, sugars, carboxylic and amino acids in model systems and in citrus fruits. *J Chromatogr A* 1149: 88–101 (2007).
37. Gall GL, DuPont MS, Mellon FA, Davis AL, Collins GJ, Verhoeyen ME and Colquhoun IJ, Characterization and content of flavonoid glycosides in genetically modified tomato (*Lycoersicon esculentum*) fruits. *J Agric Food Chem* 51: 2438–2446 (2003).
38. Gardana C, Guarnieri S, Riso P, Simonetti P and Porrini M, Flavanone plasma pharmacokinetics from blood orange juice in human subjects. *Brit J Nutr* 98: 165–172 (2007).
39. Giusti MM, Rodríguez-Saona LE, Griffin D and Wrolstad RE, Electrospray and tandem mass spectroscopy as tools for anthocyanin characterization. *J Agric Food Chem* 47: 4657–4664 (1999).
40. Gomez-Prieto MS, Caja MM, Herraiz M and Santa-Maria G, Supercritical fluid extraction of all-*trans*-lycopene from tomato. *J Agric Food Chem* 51: 3–7 (2003).
41. Goodwin TW, Biosynthesis of carotenoids: An overview, *Method Enzymol* 214: 330–340 (1992).
42. Griffith AP and Collison MW, Improved methods for the extraction and analysis of isoflavones from soy-containing foods and nutritional supplements by reversed-phase high performance liquid chromatography and liquid chromatography–mass spectrometry. *J Chromatogr A* 913: 397–413 (2001).
43. Grotewold E, The challenges of moving chemicals within and out of cells: Insights into the transport of plant natural products. *Planta* 219: 906–909 (2004).
44. Guadalupe Z, Soldevilla A, Saenz-Navajas MP and Ayestaran B, Analysis of polymeric phenolics in red wines using different techniques combined with gel permeation chromatography fractionation. *J Chromatogr A* 1112: 112–120 (2006).
45. Gueguen S, Herbeth B, Siest G and Leroy P, An isocratic liquid chromatographic method with diode-array detection for the simultaneous determination of α-tocopherol, retinol, and five carotenoids in human serum. *J Chromatogr Sci* 40: 69–76 (2002).
46. Hadden WL, Watkins RH, Levy LW, Regalado E, Rivadeneira DM, van Breemen RB and Schwartz SJ, Carotenoid composition of marigold (*Tagetes erecta*) flower extract used as nutritional supplement. *J Agric Food Chem* 47: 4189–4194 (1999).

47. Hakkinen SH, Karenlampi SO, Heinonen IM, Mykkanen HM and Torronen AR, Content of the flavonols quercetin, myricetin, and kaempferol in 25 edible berries. *J Agric Food Chem* 47: 2274–2279 (1999).
48. Harborne JB, General procedures and measurement of total phenolics. In: *Methods in plant biochemistry*, vol. 1, Ed., Harborne JB, Academic Press, San Diego, CA, pp. 1–28 (1989).
49. Harborne JB, Ed., *The flavonoids: Advances in research since 1986*, Chapman & Hall, London (1996).
50. Harborne JB and Williams CA, Advances in flavonoid research since 1992. *Phytochemistry* 55: 481–504 (2000).
51. Hassimotto NMA, Genovese MI and Lajolo FM, Identification and characterization of anthocyanins from wild mulberry (*Morus nigra* L.) growing in Brazil. *Food Sci Tech Int* 13: 17–25 (2007).
52. Hertog MGL, Hollman PCH and Venema DP, Optimization of a quantitative HPLC determination of potentially anticarcinogenic flavonoids in vegetables and fruits. *J Agric Food Chem* 40: 1591–1598 (1992).
53. Hertog MGL and Hollman PCH, Potential health effects of the dietary flavonols quercetin. *Eur J Clin Nutr* 50: 63–71 (1996).
54. Hollman PCH, van Trijp JMP and Buysman MNCP, Fluorescence detection of flavonols in HPLC by postcolumn chelation with aluminum. *Anal Chem* 68: 3511–3515 (1996).
55. Hollman PCH, van Trijp JMP, Buysman MNCP, Gaag MS, Mengelers MJB, de Vries JHM and Katan MB, Relative bioavailability of the antioxidant flavonoid quercetin from various foods in man. *FEBS Lett* 418: 152–156 (1997).
56. Hollman PCH and Arts ICW, Flavonols, flavones and flavanols—Nature, occurrence and dietary burden. *J Sci Food Agric* 80: 1081–1093 (2000).
57. Isaksen M and Francis GW, Reversed-phase thin-layer chromatography of carotenoids. *J Chromatogr* 355: 358–362 (1986).
58. Jamshidi A, Adjvadi M and Husain SW, Determination of kaempferol and quercetin in an extract of *Ginkgo biloba* leaves by high-performance thin-layer chromatography (HPTLC). *J Planar Chromatogr* 13: 57–59 (2000).
59. Justesen U, Negative atmospheric pressure chemical ionization low-energy collision activation mass spectrometry for the characterization of flavonoids in extracts of fresh herbs. *J Chromatogr A* 902: 369–379 (2000).
60. Khachik F, Beecher GR and Whittaker NF, Separation, identification, and quantification of the major carotenoid and chlorophyll constituents in extracts of several green vegetables by liquid chromatography. *J Agric Food Chem* 34: 603–616 (1986).
61. Khachik F, Steck A and Pfander H, Isolation and structural elucidation of (13Z,13'Z,3R,3'R,6'R)-lutein from marigold flowers, kale, and human plasma. *J Agric Food Chem* 47: 455–461 (1999).
62. Khallouki F, Haubner R, Hull WE, Erben G, Spiegelhalder B, Bartsch H and Owen RW, Isolation, purification and identification of ellagic acid derivatives, catechins, and procyanidins from the root bark of *Anisophyllea dichostyla* R. Br. *Food Chem Toxicol* 45: 472–485 (2007).
63. Klejdus B, Lojkova L, Lapcik O, Koblovska J and Kuban V, Supercritical fluid extraction of isoflavones from biological samples with ultra-fast high-performance liquid chromatography/mass spectrometry. *J Sep Sci* 28: 1334–1346 (2005).
64. Knekt P, Kumpulainen K, Jarvinen R, Rissanen H, Hellovaara M, Reunanen A, Hakulinen T and Aromaa A, Flavonoid intake and risk of chronic disease. *Am J Clin Nutr* 76: 560–568 (2002).

65. Koh E and Mitchell AE, Urinary isoflavone excretion in Korean adults: Comparisons of fermented soybean paste and unfermented soy flour. *J Sci Food Agric* 87: 2112–2120 (2007).

66. Kosir IJ, Lapornik B, Andrensek S, Wondra AG, Vrhovsek U and Kidric J, Identification of anthocyanins in wines by liquid chromatography, liquid chromatography–mass spectrometry and nuclear magnetic resonance. *Anal Chim Acta* 513: 277–282 (2004).

67. Kozminski R and Brett AMO, Reversed-phase high-performance liquid chromatography with electrochemical detection of anthocyanins. *Anal Lett* 39: 2687–2697 (2006).

68. Krause M and Galensa R, High-performance liquid chromatography of diastereomeric flavavone glycosides in *Citrus* on a β-cyclodextrin-bonded stationary phase (Cyclobond I). *J Chromatogr* 588: 41–45 (1991).

69. Kuskoski EM, Vega JM, Rios JJ, Fett R, Troncoso AM and Asuero AG, Characterization of anthocyanins from the fruits of Bajuacu (*Eugenia unbelliflora* Berg). *J Agric Food Chem* 51: 5450–5454 (2003).

70. Lacker T, Strohschein S and Albert K, Separation and identification of various carotenoids by C_{30} reversed-phase high-performance liquid chromatography coupled to UV and atmospheric pressure chemical ionization mass spectrometric detection. *J Chromatogr A* 854: 37–44 (1999).

71. Larger PJ, Jones AD and Dacombe C, Separation of tea polyphenols using micellar electrokinetic chromatography with diode array detection. *J Chromatogr A* 799: 309–320 (1998).

72. Lee MJ, Wang ZU, Li H, Chen L, Sun Y, Gobbo S, Balentine DA and Yang CS, Analysis of plasma and urinary tea polyphenols in human subjects. *Cancer Epidemiol Biomarker Prev* 4: 393–399 (1995).

73. Lee BL and Ong CN, Comparative analysis of tea catechins and theaflavins by high-performance liquid chromatography and capillary electrophoresis. *J Chromatogr A* 881: 439–447 (2000).

74. Lee MT and Chen BH, Separation of lycopene and its *cis* isomers by liquid chromatography. *Chromatographia* 54: 613–617 (2001).

75. Li X, Xiao H, Liang X, Shi D and Liu J, LC-MS/MS determination of naringin, hesperidin and neohesperidin in rat serum after orally administrating the decoction of *Bulpleurum falcatum* L. and *Fractus aurantii*. *J Pharm Biomed Anal* 34: 159–166 (2004).

76. Lin YY, Ng KJ and Yang S, Characterization of flavonoids by liquid chromatography–tandem mass chromatography. *J Chromatogr* 629: 389–393 (1993).

77. Lommen A, Godejohann M, Venema DP, Hollman PCH and Spraul M, Application of directly coupled HPLC-NMR-MS to the identification and confirmation of quercetin glycosides and phloretin glycosides in apple peel. *Anal Chem* 72: 1793–1797 (2000).

78. Machlin LJ, Critical assessment of epidemiological data concerning the impact of antioxidant nutrients on cancer and cardiovascular disease. *Critical Rev Food Sci Nutr* 35: 41–50 (1995).

79. Males Z and Medic-Saric M, Optimization of TLC analysis of flavonoids and phenolic acids of *Helleborus atrorubens* Waldst. et Kit. *J Pharm Biomed Anal* 24: 353–359 (2001).

80. Maoka T, Fujiwara Y, Hashimoto K and Akimoto N, Characterization of epoxy carotenoids by fast atom bombardment collision-induced dissociation MS/MS. *Lipids* 39: 179–183 (2004).

81. Medic-Saric M, Jasprica I, Smolcic-Bubalo A and Mornar A, Optimization of chromatographic conditions in thin layer chromatography of flavonoids and phenolic acids. *Croatica Chemica Acta* 77: 361–366 (2004).

82. Melendez-Martínez AJ, Vicario IM and Heredia FJ, A routine high-performance liquid chromatography method for carotenoids determination in ultrafrozen orange juices. *J Agric Food Chem* 51: 4219–4224 (2003).

83. Merken HM, Merken CD and Beecher GR, Kinetics method for the quantitation of antho-cyanidins, flavonols, and flavones in foods. *J Agric Food Chem* 49: 2727–2732 (2001).

84. Milbury PE, Chen CY, Dolnikowski GG and Blumberg JB, Determination of flavonoids and phenolics and their distribution in almonds. *J Agric Food Chem* 54: 5027–5033 (2006).

85. Mitchell AE, Hong YJ, Koh E, Barrett DM, Bryant DE, Denison RF and Kaffka S, Ten-year comparison of the influence of organic and conventional crop management practices on the content of flavonoids in tomatoes. *J Agric Food Chem* 55: 6154–6159 (2007).

86. Mullen W, Boitier A, Stewart AJ and Crozier A, Flavonoid metabolites in human plasma and urine after the consumption of red onions: Analysis by liquid chromatography with photodiode array and full scan tandem mass spectrometric detection. *J Chromatogr A* 1058: 163–168 (2004).

87. Murphy P, Barua K and Hauck CC, Solvent extraction selection in the determination of isoflavones in soy foods. *J Chromatogr B* 777: 129–138 (2002).

88. Nijveldt RJ, van Nood E, van Hoorn DEC, Boelens PG, van Norren K and van Leeuwen PAM, Flavonoids: A review of probable mechanisms of action and potential applica-tions. *Am J Clin Nutr* 74: 418–425 (2001).

89. Onyilagha O and Grotewold E, The biology and structural distribution of surface fla-vonoids. *Recent Res Devel Plant Sci* 2: 53–71 (2004).

90. Pereira CAM, Yariwake JH, Lancas FM, Wauters JN, Tits M and Angenot L, A HPTLC densitometric determination of flavonoids from *Passiflora alata, P. edulis, P. incarnate* and *P. caerulea* and comparison with HPLC method. *Phytochem Anal* 15: 241–248 (2004).

91. Pfander H and Riesen R, Chromatography: Part IV. High-performance liquid chroma-tography. In: *Carotenoids,* vol. 1A, Eds., Britton G, Liaaen-Jensen S and Pfander H, Birkhauser Verlag, Basel, pp. 145–190 (1995).

92. Pietta P, Flavonoids as antioxidants. *J Nat Prod* 63: 1035–1042 (2000).

93. Prasain JK, Jones K, Kirk M, Wilson L, Smith-Johnson M, Weaver C and Barnes S, Profiling and quantification of isoflavonoids in kudzu dietary supplements by high-performance liquid chromatography and electrospray ionization tandem mass spectrom-etry. *J Agric Food Chem* 51: 4213–4218 (2003).

94. Rao RN, Alvi SN and Rao BN, Preparative isolation and characterization of some minor impurities of astaxanthin by high-performance liquid chromatography. *J Chromatogr A* 1076: 189–192 (2005).

95. Rauha JP, Vuorela H and Kostiainen R, Effect of eluent on the ionization efficiency of flavonoids by ion spray, atmospheric pressure chemical ionization, and atmospheric pressure photoionization mass spectrometry. *J Mass Spectrom* 36: 1269–1280 (2001).

96. Reich E, Schibli A, Widmer V, Jorns R, Wolfram E and DeBatt A, HPTLC methods for identification of green tea and green tea extract. *J Liq Chrom Rel Technol* 29: 2141–2151 (2006).

97. Rentel C, Strohschein S, Albert K and Bayer E, Silver-plated vitamins: A method of detecting tocopherols and carotenoids in LC/ESI-MS coupling. *Anal Chem* 70: 4394–4400 (1998).

98. Rijke E, Zafra-Gomez A, Ariese F, Brinkman UAT and Gooijer C, Determination of isoflavone glucoside malonates in *Trifolium pratense* L. (red clover) extracts: Quantifi-cation and stability studies. *J Chromatogr A* 932: 55–64 (2001).

99. Satterfield M, Black DM and Brodbelt JS, Detection of the isoflavone aglycones genistein and daidzein in urine using solid-phase microextraction–high-performance liquid chromatography–electrospray ionization mass spectrometry. *J Chromatogr B* 759: 33–41 (2001).

100. Schieber A, Keller P, Streker P, Klaiber I and Carle R, Detection of isorhamnetin gly-cosides in extracts of apples (*Malus domestic* acv. "Brettacher") by HPLC-PDA and HPLC-APCI-MS/MS. *Phytochem Anal* 13: 87–94 (2002).

101. Schierle J, Bretzel W, Bühler I, Faccin N, Hess D, Steiner K and Schüep W, Content and iso-meric ratio of lycopene in food and human blood plasma. *Food Chem* 59: 459–465 (1997).

102. Schroeter H, Heiss C, Balzer J, Kleinbongard P, Keen C, Hollenberg N, Sies H, Kwik-Urib C, Schimitz H and Kelm M, (–)-Epicatechin mediates beneficial effects of flavonol rich cocoa on vascular function in humans. *Proc Natl Acad Sci USA* 103: 1024–1029 (2006).

103. Setchell KDR, Welsh MB and Lim CK, High-performance liquid chromatographic anal-ysis of phytoestrogens in soy protein preparations with ultraviolet, electrochemical and thermospray mass spectrometric detection. *J Chromatogr* 386: 315–323 (1987).

104. Soleas GJ, Yan J and Goldberg DM, Ultrasensitive assay for three polyphenols (cat-echin, quercetin and resveratrol) and their conjugates in biological fluids utilizing gas chromatography with mass selective detection. *J Chromatogr B* 757: 161–172 (2001).

105. Stamp N, Out of the quagmire of plant hypotheses. *Q Rev Biol* 78: 23–55 (2003).

106. Toor RK, Savage GP and Lister CE, Seasonal variations in the antioxidant composition of greenhouse grown tomatoes. *J Food Comp Anal* 19: 1–10 (2006).

107. Vallejo F, Tomas-Barberan FA and Ferreres F, Characterization of flavonols in broccoli (*Brassica oleracea* L. var. *italica*) by liquid chromatography–UV diode array detection–electrospray ionization mass spectrometry. *J Chromatogr A* 1054: 181–193 (2004).

108. van Acker SA, Tromp MN, Haenen GR, van der Vijgh WJ and Bast A, Flavonoids as a scavengers of nitric oxide radical. *Biochem Biophys Res Comm* 214: 755–759 (1995).

109. van Breemen RB, Xu X, Viana MA, Chen L, Stacewicz-Sapuntzakis M, Duncan C, Bowen PE and Sharifi R, Liquid chromatography–mass spectrometry of *cis*- and all-*trans*-lycopene in human serum and prostate tissue after dietary supplementation with tomato sauce. *J Agric Food Chem* 50: 2214–2219 (2002).

110. Vanamala J, Reddivari L, Yoo KS, Pike LM and Patil BS, Variation in the content of bioactive flavonoids in different brands of orange and grapefruit juices. *J Food Comp Anal* 19: 157–166 (2006).

111. Vovk I, Simonovska B and Vuorela H, Separation of eight selected flavan-3-ols on cel-lulose thin-layer chromatographic plates. *J Chromatogr A* 1077: 188–194 (2005).

112. Vrhovsek U, Rigo A, Tonon D and Mattivi F, Quantitation of polyphenols in different apple varieties. *J Agric Food Chem* 52: 6532–6538 (2004).

113. Wang CY, Huang HY, Kuo KL and Hsieh YZ, Analysis of *Puerariae radix* and its medic-inal preparations by capillary electrophoresis. *J Chromatogr A* 802: 225–231 (1998).

114. Waridel P, Wolfender JL, Ndjoko K, Hobby KR, Major HJ and Hostettmann K, Evalua-tion of quadrupole time-of-flight tandem mass spectrometry and ion-trap multiple-stage mass spectrometry for the differentiation of C-glycosidic flavonoid isomers. *J Chro-matogr A* 926: 29–41 (2001).

115. Williamson G and Manach C, Bioavailability and bioefficacy of polyphenols in humans. II. Review of 93 intervention studies. *Am J Clin Nutr* 81: 243S–255S (2005).

116. Wollgast J and Anklam E, Review on polyphenols in *Theobroma cacao*: Changes in composition during the manufacture of chocolate and methodology for identification and quantification. *Food Res Int* 33: 423–447 (2000).

CHAPTER 4

Anti-inflammatory Botanicals
A Case Study of Genetic Screens as Part of a Pharmacogenomic Approach

Moul Dey, Igor Belolipov, Salohutdin Zakirov, Anarbek Akimaliev, Jamin Akimaliev, Ishimby Sodonbekov, and Ilya Raskin

CONTENTS

INTRODUCTION

Pharmaceuticals developed from natural and synthetic sources, based on single active ingredients, are usually called new chemical entities (NCEs). Inflammatory diseases are currently treated with steroidal and nonsteroidal anti-inflammatory drugs (NSAIDs), most of which belong to the class of NCEs [1,2]. Yearly, more than 80 million prescriptions are written worldwide to treat inflammatory diseases, in addition to the over-the-counter (OTC) sales [3,4]. One in seven Americans is likely to receive an NSAID for a chronic rheumatologic disorder [3,5], often on a daily basis. However, NCE drugs are becoming increasingly unpopular due to the significant negative side effects associated with their continuous use [1,2]. This, coupled with demands of the ever growing world population, calls for the development of novel drugs that are effective and safe for long-term use.

A World Health Organization (WHO) survey indicated that about 70–80% of the world's populations use nonconventional medicine—mainly herbals—as part of their primary healthcare [6]. In recent years, the United States also witnessed an increased growth in popularity of OTC health foods, nutraceuticals, and medicinal products from plants or other natural sources. About 62% of the U.S. population during the year 2002 used some form of complementary and alternative medicine (CAM) other than megavitamins [7]. Plants synthesize bewildering arrays of organic molecules with functions that have puzzled generations of natural product chemists. Not surprisingly, in the areas of cancer, infectious, and inflammatory diseases that are mechanistically linked, about 60–75% of the new drugs developed during 1983–1994 were based on naturally occurring compounds [8,9]. This is in spite of the fact that a majority of the phytochemicals produced by 250,000 plant species of the world still remains unexplored [10]. On the other hand, purely synthetic approaches such as combinatorial chemistry and computational drug designs have not achieved its often touted potential during the past 20 years [11]. Therefore, seeking to investigate the vast chemodiversity among natural resources such as plant species seems a rational proposition [10,12].

It is possible that the evolutionary significance of a large number of phytochemicals present in each plant lies in their complex, mutually potentiating effects that provide protection against diverse pests, pathogens, and herbivores. Modern medicine has only recently learned how pathogens and cancer cells can develop quick resistance to single-ingredient drugs, and that the administration of complex drug cocktails can circumvent or delay such resistance buildup. Plants may have learned such strategy very early in their evolution. However, efficient identification, study, and development of such multicomponent botanicals could not be achieved in the past by using high-throughput screening (HTS) methods [10,13]. HTS methods are usually adapted to test a single active ingredient, which is why development of NCEs was favored over natural products during the past decades. Hence, revisiting the screening and developmental approaches for botanicals in the postgenomic era is a necessary and timely consideration. A case study for screening anti-inflammatory botanicals (Dey et al., in press) [13a] and strategies (Figure 4.1) to further develop the identified hits into advanced therapeutic leads are discussed below. For the initial screens, cell-based gene expression assays were used that will fit into the pharmacogenomic drug developmental scheme also described.

PHARMACOGENOMICS IS A NASCENT FIELD

The Human Genome Project has provided the foundation for understanding health and disease at the genetic level. Pharmacogenomics (pharmacological genomics) is an integrative system biology that uses tools and concepts from pharmacology, molecular biology, genetics and genomics (http://genomics.energy.gov/). It is believed that differences in responses to medications may occur among individuals whose genetic makeups vary due to single nucleotide polymorphisms (SNPs) [14], gene copy number variations (CNVs) [15], or other widespread dissimilarities. For example, anti-inflammatory drugs targeting cytokine signaling pathways will show

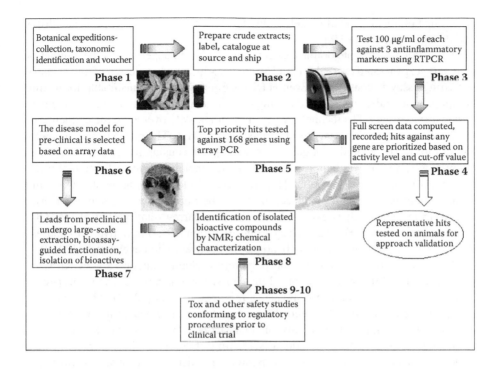

Figure 4.1 Proposed development of anti-inflammatory botanicals: a pharmacological paradigm.

variable efficacies based on the SNPs in cytokine encoding genes [16]. Considering such genetic differences, pharmacogenomics holds the promise that drugs might one day be tailor-made for individuals, adapting to each person's own genetic makeup. This can also lead to the characterization of powerful existing drugs with a particular emphasis on how to reduce recurrence of any known adverse drug reactions [17].

Cells respond to therapeutic cues by activating signal-transduction pathways that drive specific patterns of gene expression. Transcriptional machineries with their numerous components play a key role in such genetic modulation. Hence, to search the possible pharmacological effect of a plant extract or to compare the mode of actions of various anti-inflammatory extracts, knowledge of the genes whose expression changes in response to the therapeutic signal is essential. Pharmacogenomics as a developing research field is still in its infancy, with new information regarding candidate genes and disease pathways being uncovered every day. Hence, there are challenges to overcome before this rapidly accumulating genomic information can be applied to understand variable drug responses. These include relating disease genes to drug response genes, precisely defining drug response phenotypes, and addressing analytic, ethical, and technological issues involved in generation and management of large data sets. Overcoming these challenges will enhance novel drug developments, including botanicals, and ultimately individualize the selection of appropriate drugs and dosages for patients [18].

Paradoxically, in spite of this nascent state of pharmacogenomics, the number of drug targets generated every day could be overwhelming when design of any primary screening assay is considered. Even HTS systems, which are unsuitable for testing complex botanicals, now face a daunting challenge against such increased numbers of new drug targets. The technology that may potentially overcome the challenge of screening against multiple targets at a time is microarray. The microarray is a powerful tool for rapid generation of gene expression profiles using living cells or tissues. Surprisingly, not many attempts to utilize this technology for identification of novel botanicals have been made so far [19]. However, lack of validation standards and quality controls presents a bottleneck in using the microarray technology for drug screening in general. It is expected that the microarray quality control (MAQC) project, a current U.S. Food and Drug Administration (FDA) initiative, will address these issues to foster its proper applications in discovery and development [20,21].

Quantitative reverse transcription polymerase chain reaction (RT–PCR)-based arrays are powerful new tools for profiling expression of genes induced from specific disease signaling cascades in response to therapeutic cues [22,23]. This emerging platform offers a balance between the specificity and reproducibility of real-time PCR and the multitarget versatility of microarrays. This platform is particularly valuable for "high content" functional screening of complex plant extracts against biological targets in living cells, tissues, and organisms. PCR-array monitors the amount of amplicon generated as the real-time reaction progresses and can profile both up- and down-regulation of a battery of genes expressed during a disease process in a simple 96-well format. Instead of a system-wide generic search for gene expressions, as in the case of microarrays, PCR array systemically targets disease pathway-specific genes. Most diseases involve more than one signaling circuit and PCR array can potentially establish the cross-talk among them. We have observed [24] that the robustness of the real-time PCR system allows it to detect the biological activity of a compound present within a complex mixture of chemicals with a comparable sensitivity when the compound is tested in its pure form. The data generated present the percent change of gene expression in response to any specific treatment, enabling quick hit prioritization.

ANTI-INFLAMMATORY BOTANICALS FROM CENTRAL ASIA

The summary of a screening work (Dey et al., in press) is presented here as a case study. Real-time gene expression assays with three genetic markers were optimized for identification of anti-inflammatory botanical hits from a large number of crude plant extracts (Table 4.1). To validate this initial approach, selected hits were tested on animals to treat anti-inflammatory conditions *in vivo*. The representative hits were effective and bioavailable in rats (Dey et al., in press). Hence, the next strategy is to test each of the priority hits against an array of 168 genes that include transmembrane receptors and kinases, other proteins residing in the cytoplasm, and

Table 4.1   Screen Summary of Anti-Inflammatory Botanicals from Central Asia

Data Set	Statistics	Notes
Number of extracts screened	1000	—
Number of plant families screened	~68	Collection from Central Asia
Number of plant species screened	~449	—
Number of hits from extracts (≥75% inhibition in at least one gene)	75 (7.5%)	—
Number of hits from species (≥75% inhibition in at least one gene)	58 (~12.9%)	—
Number of families producing hits (≥75% inhibition, at least one gene)	21 (~30.8%)	—
Hits for COX2 (≥75%; ≥50%)	8 (0.8%); 49 (4.9%)	See Figure 4.2
Hits for IL1β (≥75%; ≥50%)	74 (7.4%); 172 (17.2%)	See Figure 4.2; one from this group validated *in vivo*
Hits for iNOS (≥75%; ≥50%)	21 (2.1%); 105 (10.5%)	See Figure 4.2
Hits for any two genes (≥75%)	12 (1.2%)	Two from this group validated *in vivo*
Hits for all three genes (≥75%)	6 (0.6%)	One from this group validated *in vivo*

transcription factors and effector molecules further downstream of the transcription machinery. These genes are representative of two well-defined and interconnected signaling cascades that are key players in inflammation and immune responses.

Inflammation is associated with various diseases such as rheumatoid arthritis, cancer, myocarditis, arteriosclerosis, bowel diseases, multiple sclerosis, asthma, and many others. While several inflammatory markers are commonly expressed during any inflammatory disorder, some are symptom specific. Therefore, the gene array data will be particularly helpful in indicating the appropriate disease model for subsequent preclinical and clinical tests. Only functional, active extracts with potentially safe and novel modes of actions may then be subjected to labor-intensive large-scale extraction, fractionation, characterization, and isolation of novel bioactive components. We believe that the strategy as described schematically in Figure 4.1 will allow efficient use of plant extracts and other natural resources toward identification of novel drug leads for human health care.

Plant materials were obtained from diverse geographic locations in two central Asian countries—Uzbekistan and Kyrgyzstan—and collected through the International Cooperative Biodiversity Group (ICBG) program of the U.S. National Institutes of Health. Monocytes play a central role in inflammation [25]. Therefore, a mouse macrophage cell line, RAW 264.7, was chosen for the cellular assay system. Bacterial lipopolysaccharide (LPS) activates monocytes by binding to cell membrane receptor complexes and induces various proinflammatory genes that are involved in adaptive as well as innate immunity-related disorders [24,26,27]. For the initial screening of 1000 crude plant extracts, we selected a cytokine interleukin 1β (IL1β) and two redox sensitive enzyme-encoding genes—inducible nitric oxide synthase (iNOS) and cyclooxygenase2—as proinflammatory markers for our screening system. These genes are strongly induced during inflammation and are responsible for its onset and maintenance. IL1β is a cytokine that acts as a signaling molecule for immune cells to coordinate the inflammatory response [28]. COX2 has drawn attention as a popular target for many modern anti-inflammatory and cancer-preventive drugs [1,2]. It is an enzyme necessary for the formation of proinflammatory prostaglandins. Nitric oxide (NO) is a short-lived free radical that mediates many physiological and pathophysiological processes, including neurotransmission and inflammation [29]. The iNOS catalyzes the conversion of L-arginine to NO and L-citrulline with oxygen and nicotinamide adenine dinucleotide phosphate (NADPH) as cosubstrates. Expression of iNOS in activated macrophages is mainly regulated at transcriptional levels, particularly by nuclear factor kappaB (NF-kB) and other mediators [25,29].

The summary of the screening data of 1000 plant extracts is presented in Table 4.1. Percent inhibition of gene expression compared to untreated control was the single variable used in screening. When treated at the concentration of 100 μg/ml, extracts showing greater than 75% inhibition (a stringent criterion) for *COX2, iNOS,* or *IL1*β were counted as hits, unless mentioned otherwise. The screening system was initially standardized and validated by dose–response tests conducted with known anti-inflammatory compounds (positive standards) such as parthenolide [30] and phenethylisothiocyanate (PEITC) [24]. It was established that the assays were comparable in their robustness and efficiency when used to detect the biological activity of pure PEITC and that of the PEITC present within a crude plant extract as a bioactive component [24].

The screening of 1000 plant extracts resulted in a 0.8% hit rate for *COX2,* 2.1% for *iNOS,* 7.4% for *IL1*β (Figure 4.2), and 0.6% for all three assays combined (Table 4.1). When data from any two out of three genes were combined, the hit rate was 1.2% (Table 4.1). Only 0.2% of the extracts showed 100% inhibition of *COX2* induction by LPS. Similarly, complete inhibition of *iNOS* and *IL1*β induction was produced by 0.3 and 0.7% of extracts, respectively. Reducing the stringency from 75 to 50% increased the number of hits to 4.9% for *COX2,* 10.5% for *iNOS,* and 17.2% for *IL1*β assays (Table 4.1). About 3.5% of extracts were cytotoxic at the tested concentration of 100

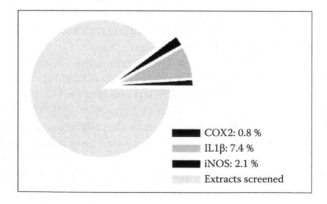

Figure 4.2   Percent hits (out of 1000 extracts) in the genetic screen.

μg/ml, yielding inconclusive data. The identified hits were further tested for their dose-dependent effects on the gene expression assays (data not shown here).

Overall, 75 out of 1000 (7.5%) extracts passed the 75% stringency requirement for at least one gene (Table 4.1). Sixty-eight plant families were screened, out of which 21 (30.8%) families containing 337 species produced 58 (12.9%) species hits (Table 4.1). The number of tested extracts was greater than the number of tested species because several plant parts from the same species were often extracted and tested (e.g., leaves and roots).

Primary screening data correlated with the *in vivo* results. Four selected hits, when tested on a carrageenan induced rat paw edema model of acute inflammation and were bioavailable and pharmacologically active, reducing swelling of the paw (data not shown here). The efficacies of the extracts were measured by calculating the reduction in swelling as compared to the vehicle-treated control. Aspirin was used as a positive control for anti-inflammatory activity. These observations validated the potential use of the hits discovered in the RT-PCR assay for the *in vivo* anti-inflammatory applications.

The ongoing studies consist of testing the identified hits in PCR arrays for determining the key genes that regulate NFkB and TLR (Toll-like receptor) signaling pathways (Figure 4.1). NFkB is the central factor controlling the transcription mechanisms involved in inflammatory and immune responses as well as in cancer [25,28]. The three genetic markers used in the primary screening have NFkB binding domains upstream of their respective promoter regions, indicating that their role in cell signaling is at least partially coordinated by this transcription factor [28].

The TLR cascade is present upstream of the NFkB pathway. Toll receptors are type I transmembrane proteins involved in various biological processes during inflammation including pathogen recognition [31]. In mammalian systems, TLRs and the receptors for any type of IL1 cytokine share a cytoplasmic motif, the Toll/IL1 receptor (TIR) domain, which is required for initiating intracellular signaling during pathogen-initiated inflammatory and immune responses [32]. Because the primary screening data indicate a trend of greater abundance of IL1β inhibitors among plant species (Table 4.1) as compared to inhibitors for the other two markers, studying this signaling cascade may reveal significant information related to the mechanisms of therapeutic actions of the identified plant products. Also, the TIR superfamily is evolutionarily conserved between mammals and insects, preserving its role in host defense [31]. Interestingly, insect pests are the main causes of plant diseases and death, against which plants have often adapted the use of secondary metabolites as part of plant defense mechanisms [10].

CONCLUSIONS

The case study discussed here has currently entered the fifth phase of the proposed developmental plan for anti-inflammatory botanicals (Figure 4.1). The experimental paradigms are based on preexisting technologies and available genetic information that resulted from genome sequencing projects. However, the overall approach suggests a complete new direction and is likely to overcome the challenge raised by the lack of scientific research–based, consistent, and reliable botanical products in the U.S. markets today. Results obtained so far are encouraging as they indicate a potential and significant improvement from the published hit rates obtained from other pharmacological screening systems and drug discovery approaches. With an average hit rate of 0.1–0.5% [11], to have a reliable screen that will minimize lead failure at later developmental stages is the biggest challenge faced by the present pharmaceutical industries; lead failure not only is counterproductive, but also results in huge economic losses [11]. On average, only 40–50% of the identified hits (0.1–0.5%) generate leads [33]. From the case study presented here, the hit rate was 7.5% with a very stringent cut-off criterion. The *in vivo* hit validation was 100%, although only a small segment of the hits were considered for this initial "proof of concept" study.

Large-scale preclinical investigations will be carried out in the near future as proposed in Figure 4.1. It is worthwhile to mention here that unlike synthetic drug hits, many of the screened plants are known to be edible, implying that they may be better tolerated in humans. Since they have been tested on complex living cells and not against isolated targets, subsequent target validations in secondary screens are not necessary. Also, hit ranking and clustering are simple and precise in contrast to a "hit or miss" qualitative assay system and are based on numerical values for gene inhibition. Together, the so-called "hit to lead challenge" [34] is expected to be substantially low. Therefore, it is possible that most of the hits will potentially become advanced therapeutic leads.

Development of botanical drug/food supplements based on genetic screens and pharmacogenomic strategy appears to have several advantages. It is likely that, on the one hand, this will minimize the causes of lead failure at a later stage, enhancing the overall productivity of the drug industry. On the other hand, matching the suitability of a drug, initially identified from genetic screens and developed based on gene array investigations with a patient's genetic profile, which is expected to be a routine procedure in the near future [35,36], will be easier. Also, the drug approval process should be facilitated as trials of such leads can be targeted for only the genetically compatible segment of the population, potentially providing greater degrees of success. Here it is necessary to mention that strict regulations should be implemented for botanical food supplements to improve batch-to-batch functional consistencies in context of active ingredients and health benefits. This will also help alleviate the present situation, where the lack of regulation promotes substantial pseudoscience to the consumer and "poisons the well" for science-based commercial products. To conclude, it is possible to develop safe and effective research-based natural products guided by rational regulatory standards, thereby validating their applications in medicine. The pharmacogenomic approach is one option worth considering for achieving such a goal.

ACKNOWLEDGMENTS

Research supported by Phytomedics, Inc. (Jamesburg, New Jersey); NIH Center for Dietary Supplements Research on Botanicals and Metabolic Syndrome, grant # 1-P50 AT002776-01; Fogarty International Center of the NIH under U01 TW006674 for the International Cooperative Biodiversity Groups; and Rutgers University.

LIST OF ABBREVIATIONS

CAM: complementary and alternative medicine
CNV: [gene] copy number variation
COX2: cyclooxygenase2
FDA: Food and Drug Administration
HTS: high-throughput screening
ICBG: International Cooperative Biodiversity Group
IL1β: interleukin1β
IL8: interleukin 8
iNOS: inducible nitric oxide synthase
LPS: lipopolysaccharide
MAQC: microarray quality control [project]
NCE: new chemical entity
NFkB: nuclear factor kappaB
NO: nitric oxide
NSAID: nonsteroidal anti-inflammatory drug
OTC: over the counter
RT-PCR: reverse transcription polymerase chain reaction
SNP: single nucleotide polymorphism
TIR: Toll/IL1 receptor
TLR: Toll-like receptor
WHO: World Health Organization

REFERENCES

1. Juni, P., Reichenbach, S., and Egger, M., COX2 inhibitors, traditional NSAIDs and the heart, *Brit. Med. J.,* 330, 1342, 2005.
2. Pathak, S.K. et al., Oxidative stress and cyclooxygenase activity in prostate carcinogenesis, targets for chemopreventive strategies, *Eur. J. Cancer*, 41(1), 61, 2005.
3. Clive, D.M. and Stoff, J.S., Renal syndromes associated with NSAIDs, *New Engl. J. Med.*, 310, 563, 1984.
4. Langman, M.J.S., Ulcer complications and NSAIDs, *Am. J. Med.*, 84 (2A), 15, 998.
5. Whelton, A. and Hamilton, C.W., NSAIDs: Effects on kidney function, *J. Clin. Pharmacol.*, 31, 588, 1991.

6. Chan, K., Some aspects of toxic contaminants in herbal medicines, *Chemosphere*, 52(9), 1361, 2003.
7. Barnes, P. et al., Complementary and alternative medicine use by U.S. adults during year 2002, *CDC Adv. Data Rep.*, 343, 2004.
8. Newman, D.J., Cragg, G.M., and Snader, K.M.J., Natural products as sources of new drugs over the period 1981–2002, *J. Nat. Prod.*, 66, 1022, 2003.
9. Newman, D.J. and Cragg, G.M., Natural products as sources of new drugs over the last 25 years, *J. Nat. Prod.*, 70, 461, 2007.
10. Raskin, I. and Ripoll, C., Can an apple a day keep the doctor away? *Curr. Pharm. Design*, 10, 3419, 2004.
11. Dove, A., Drug screening—Beyond the bottleneck, *Nat. Biotechnol.*, 17(9), 859, 1999.
12. Raskin, I. et al., Plants and human health in the 21st century, *Trends Biotechnol.*, 20, 522, 2002.
13. Lila, M.A. and Raskin, I., Health-related interactions of phytochemicals, *J. Food Sci.*, 70, R20, 2005.
13a. Dey, M. et al., Natural product screen using pro-inflammatory gene transcription assay. *Phytotherapy Research*, in press.
14. Delrieu, O. and Bowman, C., Visualizing gene determinants of disease in drug discovery, *Pharmacogenomics*, 3, 311, 2006.
15. Lee, J.A. and Lupski, J.R., Genomic rearrangements and gene copy-number alterations as a cause of nervous system disorders, *Neuron*, 52(1), 103, 2006.
16. Hollegaard, M.V. and Bidwel, J.L., Cytokine gene polymorphism in human disease: Online databases (supplement 3), *Genes Immun.*, 4, 269, 2006.
17. Evans, W.E. and McLeod, H.L., Pharmacogenomics—Drug disposition, drug targets, and side effects, *New Engl. J. Med.*, 348, 358, 2003.
18. Roden, D.M. et al., Pharmacogenomics: Challenges and opportunities, *Ann. Intern. Med.*, 145(10), 749, 2006.
19. Hudson, J. and Altamirano, M., The application of DNA microarrays (gene arrays) to the study of herbal medicines, *J. Ethnopharmacol.*, 108, 2, 2006.
20. Shi, L. et al., MAQC Consortium. The MicroArray Quality Control (MAQC) project shows inter- and intraplatform reproducibility of gene expression measurements, *Nat. Biotechnol.*, 9, 1151, 2006.
21. Strauss, E., Arrays of hope, *Cell*, 127(4), 657, 2006.
22. Singh, S. et al., Molecular profiles of mitogen activated protein kinase signaling pathways in orofacial development birth defects, *Res. Clin. Mol. Teratol.*, 79, 35, 2007.
23. Gude, N. et al., Akt promotes increased cardiomyocyte cycling and expansion of the cardiac progenitor cell population, *Circ. Res.*, 99, 381, 2006.
24. Dey, M. et al., Transcriptional modulation and *in vivo* anti-inflammatory activity of a seed preparation containing phenethylisothiocyanate, *J. Pharmacol. Exp. Ther.*, 317(1), 326, 2006.
25. Li, Q., Withoff, S., and Verma, I.M., Inflammation-associated cancer, NF-kappaB is the lynchpin, *Trends Immunol.*, 26(6), 318, 2005.
26. Gerhauser, C. et al., Mechanism-based *in vitro* screening of potential cancer chemopreventive agents, *Mutat. Res.*, 523, 163, 2003.
27. Rose, P. et al., β-phenylethyl and 8-methylsulphinyloctyl isothiocyanates constituents of watercress suppress LPS induced production of nitric oxide and prostaglandin E2 in RAW 2647 macrophages, *Nitric Oxide*, 12(4), 237, 2005.
28. Krakauer, T., Molecular therapeutic targets in inflammation, cyclooxygenase and NFκβ, *Curr. Drug Targets*, 3(3), 317, 2004.

29. Nathan, C. and Xie, Q.W., Nitric oxide synthases: Roles, tolls, and controls, *Cell*, 78(6), 915, 1994.

30. Kwok, B.H. et al., The anti-inflammatory natural product parthenolide from the medicinal herb Feverfew directly binds to and inhibits IkappaB kinase, *Chem. Biol.*, 8, 759, 2001.

31. Dunne, A. and O'Neill, L.A., The interleukin-1 receptor/Toll-like receptor superfamily: Signal transduction during inflammation and host defense, *Sci STKE*, 25, 2003(171), 2003.

32. Martin, M.U. and Wesche, H., Summary and comparison of the signaling mechanisms of the Toll/interleukin-1 receptor family, *Biochim. Biophys. Acta*, 1592(3), 265, 2002.

33. Fox, S. et al., High-throughput screening: Update on practices and success, *J. Biomol. Screen*, 11(7), 864, 2006.

34. Keseru, G.M. and Makara, G.M., Hit discovery and hit-to-lead approaches, *Drug Discov. Today*, 11(15), 741, 2006.

35. Hodgson, J. and Marshall A., Pharmacogenomics: Will the regulators approve? *Nat. Biotechnol.*, 16, 243, 1998.

36. Pistoi, S., Facing your genetic destiny, part II, *Sci. Am.*, Feb 25, 2002. (http://www.sciam.com/article.cfm?id=facing-your-genetic-desti-2002-02-188.page=2)

CHAPTER 5

Characteristics and Functions of Lutein and Zeaxanthin within the Human Retina

Billy R. Hammond, Jr. and Lisa M. Renzi

CONTENTS

THE PHYSICAL CHARACTERISTICS OF MACULAR PIGMENT

Physical Characteristics

The composition of the macular pigment (MP) was first established by Nobel Laureate George Wald,[1] who used a psychophysical method to noninvasively measure the spectral absorption characteristics of the yellow pigments situated within the central retina (see Figure 5.1). Based on the shape of their absorption spectra, Wald concluded that the pigments were xanthophyllic carotenoids. Approximately 40 years later, Bone, Landrum, and Tarsis[2] definitively identified these macular pigments as the specific xanthophylls (3R,3′R,6′R)-lutein (L) and (3R,3′R)-zeaxanthin

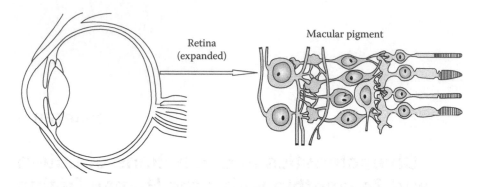

Figure 5.1   A schematic showing the neural retina lining the back of the eye and the expanded retina on the right with the macular pigments in the inner layers.

(Z). This same group (Bone et al.[3]) later identified a stereoisomer they termed (3R,3'S)-mesozeaxanthin (MZ). Z is commonly found in the diet and serum but MZ is not.[4] This observation led Bone and Landrum to conclude that MZ was converted from L within the retina itself. This conversion appears to occur in the central retina since MZ does not appear to be found beyond about 4 mm from the center.[5]

Together, L, Z, and MZ form the macular pigments. These short-wave light-absorbing pigments are obtained entirely through dietary intake of L- and Z-containing foods[6] and, due to their more recent appearance on the market, through nutritional supplements. Once ingested, L and Z are incorporated into lipid micelles within the gut and are transported to the liver for further packaging into lipoproteins.[7] High-density lipoproteins (HDLs) and, to a lesser extent, low-density and very low-density lipoproteins (LDLs and VLDLs, respectively) transport L and Z to numerous tissues within the body, including the retina.[8] Bernstein et al.[9] and Yemelyanov et al.[10] originally identified several proteins that could serve as binding sites for L and Z, including the protein tubulin, which forms part of the microtubule network that composes the cytoskeleton of cone axons. Crabtree et al.,[11] using molecular modeling, confirmed that L and Z are bound to the protein tubulin. Other potential binding proteins within the retina may include the Pi isoform of glutathione S-transferase, which may be specific for Z,[12] although this result has not been confirmed. L and Z and their isomers are the only carotenoids normally found within the eye (except under conditions of megadosing).[3,13]

Within the eye, L and Z are found at their highest concentration in the inner layers of the central retina of nonhuman primates, where they peak sharply in the very center of the macula (i.e., the fovea) and decline rapidly with eccentricity.[2] Psychophysical studies on humans[14,15] have confirmed this basic spatial pattern. For most subjects, an exponential decline with eccentricity explains the spatial density of the pigments across the retina with a relatively high degree of accuracy ($r^2 > 90\%$) (see Figure 5.2). Although most dense in the macular (hence the term "macular pigments"), L and Z have been identified at low concentrations throughout the tissues of the eye[16] (e.g., rod outer segments, subretinal fluid, retinal pigment epithelium (RPE), iridial tissue, ciliary body, supra-orbital fat) and visual pathways[17] (e.g., occipital

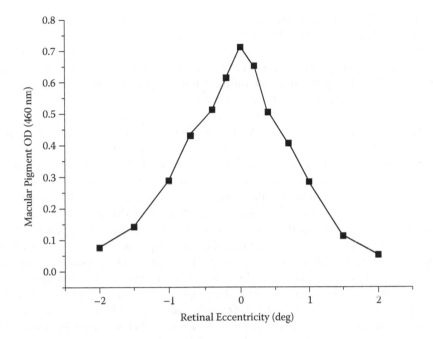

Figure 5.2 MP density measured at peak absorbance along the horizontal meridian using heterochromatic flicker photometry on one subject.

cortex). This somewhat ubiquitous and relatively exclusive presence within the visual system implies that L and Z play a special role in vision.

Variability in Macular Pigment Density

Measurement Issues

Unlike most other nutrients embedded within tissue, MP can be measured non-invasively and *in vivo*. The ability to measure these pigments in this manner has provided a powerful and unique tool for studying their characteristics within the living eye. For example, large studies (e.g., Ciulla et al., $n = 280$[18]; Hammond and Caruso-Avery, $n = 217$[19]) have found that MP varies by over a factor of 10 across individuals. Subjects have been identified with near zero levels* and levels so high that they screen a substantial portion of the short-wave end of the visible spectrum.

---

* Based on anatomical studies, we can conclude that it is very unlikely that subjects exist with no L and Z within their retinas. Although it is somewhat common to report zero MP levels in the literature, the determination of zero is made based on calculations derived from relative stimulus conditions used within the study. All retinal L and Z are derived from the diet[5] and L, for instance, is a relatively ubiquitous nutrient. No macular pigment within the retina would imply no L and Z within the diet for a relatively long period (analogous to the controlled diet study of Malinow et al.[93]). This occurrence is certainly possible but would be very rare in developed countries. Individuals with very low intake (e.g., from impoverished countries), however, might be expected to have only trace amounts of L and Z within their retinas. An alternative hypothesis is discussed later (see "Genetics and Heritability").

Such variability is apparent very early in life. For example, retinal L and Z also vary by a factor of more than 10 in the infant retina,[20] which is probably due to variation in the amount of L and Z present in breast milk and infant formula.[21] The visual system compensates for this large variation in the screening of light across the retina (e.g., from 0 to 1.6 OD (optical density) within 2 mm[14]) by increasing gain specifically within the yellow-blue color opponent system.[22,23]

Like most areas of science, a vigorous debate surrounds the issue of how best to measure MP. A number of noninvasive methods have been used, including psychophysics,[24] autofluorescence (AF),[25] fundus reflectometry (RF),[26] and Raman spectroscopy (RS).[27] Generally speaking, all of these methods appear to be somewhat reliable, although some differences exist based on the specific conditions used by a given laboratory and the population tested. Most measurement artifacts increase with age and ocular disease.[28] It is also true that all of the methods suffer from limitations and confounds that are only occasionally the same between methods. For example, many of the methods must dilate the pupil (RF, AF), often more than 7 mm (RS[29]), and/or bleach nearly all of the photopigments by using very intense light (e.g., up to 6.9 log Tds (Troland second) under conditions of "prolonged viewing"[30]). Psychophysical methods are difficult to use on subjects with visual acuity that cannot be corrected to at least 20/60 and/or are physically infirm. (Most of the methods, both physical and psychophysical, require good acuity since fixation is necessary.) Psychophysical techniques, AF, and RF are based on a relative comparison to a peripheral site (where MP is optically immeasurable), which acts as a reference to correct for confounding by the anterior media.

The exception is RS, which is based on the analysis of an absolute signal arising directly from the carotenoids themselves (i.e., elastic back-scattered light). This creates serious confounding by the anterior media and an attenuation of the signal based on the fact that the laser cannot penetrate past about 0.30 optical density units due to self-screening (see the review by Hammond and Wooten[31]). For example, when comparing MP measured using RS and AF, the overall relation is relatively strong ($r = 0.73$ from Figure 18 of Sharifzadeh et al.[30]). When considering only those values above 0.30 OD, however, the two methods do not correlate ($n = 22$, $p < 0.12$).[30] The validity of most of the methods can be confirmed by comparing the shape of the measured values with the shape of the *ex vivo* spectrum of L and Z.[31] The heterochromatic flicker photometry (HFP), RF, and AF methods have been validated using this type of evaluation and have been shown to be significantly correlated with each other.[32]

Determinants of MP Density

Perhaps one of the more striking and meaningful features of the macular pigments is their wide variation across subjects. A number of studies have been done with the aim of identifying what factors are responsible for such large individual differences. Clearly, differences in the dietary intake of L and Z explain a large proportion of the variance (the pigments cannot be synthesized de novo). This has been shown by examining the cross-sectional relations among MP, diet, and serum L and Z and through supplementation studies. Correlational studies have found relatively moderate relationships between MP and dietary intake of L and Z (e.g., Curran-Celentano et al.[33] [$r = 0.25$, $n = 280$] and Hammond et al.[34] [$r = 0.29$ in healthy adult males, $r = 0.07$ in healthy adult females, $n = 88$]). It is probably the case, however, that these relationships are underestimated due to difficulties in accurately quantifying dietary intake over time, the labile nature of the measures (e.g., serum L and Z are probably strongly influenced by recent dietary behavior, whereas MP probably reflects more long-term intake), and measurement error.[24] Nonetheless, supplementation studies (albeit short term) have also shown that the relationship is not strong and tends to be quite variable. Some subjects appear to show strong increases in MP, whereas others do not (so-called retinal nonresponders[35]).* Given the variability of response rates to supplementation and the relatively weak associations between dietary intake of L and Z and MP, we can safely conclude that there are other factors that influence MP density within the retina. The nondietary determinants that have been studied include sex, iris color, obesity, age, tobacco use, and disease status (reviewed by Mares-Perlman et al.[6]; Krinsky et al.[36]; and, more recently, Beatty et al.[37]). Relative to disease status, the effects of cystic fibrosis,[38] diabetes,[39,40] inherited retinal degenerations,[41,42] and macular degeneration (for a recent review, see Whitehead et al.[43]) have been studied. The relative importance of the various determinants of MPOD (macular pigment optical density) is not clear. For example, one question is whether MPOD decreases with age in a manner that is not tied to simple sampling differences. It is reasonable to question, for example, if MP density changes due to some underlying biological process analogous to the yellowing of the crystalline lens. Several groups have argued in favor of an age decrease (e.g., Gellermann et al.[44] and Nolan et al.[45]), suggesting that the pigments might be depleted due to decreased dietary intake in older groups, increased oxidant load, etc.[45,46] Others have argued against an age decrease (e.g., Hammond et al.,[28] Ciulla and Hammond,[47] and Berendschot and van Norren[48]), suggesting that methodological confounds are responsible for most of the age decline reported by the other groups.[28] As noted by Berendschot and van Norren,[48] the bulk of the studies that have evaluated age as a determinant have not found age declines.

What we can say is that the previously mentioned determinants, including age, appear to be clinically meaningful. For example, the personal characteristics that have been studied (e.g., dietary intake, sex, iris color, age, smoking status) have also been identified as risk factors for age-related macular degeneration (for a review, see Hammond and Johnson[49]). Typically, those factors that appear to be related to higher MP are related to lower risk and vice versa. This confluence is meaningful given the notion that MP protects the retina from damage due to light and oxygen (the protection hypothesis discussed later).

* The terms "retinal responder" and "nonresponder" were introduced by Hammond et al.[35] to reflect differences in the magnitude of MP increases that resulted from dietary supplementation. Obviously, the term "nonresponse" only refers to that response seen within the context of the study. So-called nonresponders obviously responded at some point in their lives or they would have no measurable amounts of MP. Retinal response to LZ supplementation is probably better regarded as reflecting a continuum of differences rather than simply two categories of response. The most that can be definitively said at this time is that there is clearly variability in response to supplementation and that the causes for these differences are not known.

Genetics and Heritability

Another issue that is not clear is how strongly genetics influences individual differences in MP density. Once absorbed through the gut, L and Z appear to be delivered to the two eyes in amounts that are highly similar for most individuals.[50] Such yoking implies that the pigments are under tight biological control, which suggests strong genetic influence. Hammond et al.[51] studied 10 identical twin pairs and found that 5 of the pairs had substantial differences in MP density, suggesting that, at a minimum, MP is not completely genetically determined. Recently, however, Liew et al.[52] conducted a more classic twin study (i.e., they compared 76 monozygotic to 74 dyzygotic twins) and found that the heritability of MP was quite strong (e.g., 0.67 and 0.85 when MP was measured using HFP and AF, respectively).

The results of Liew et al., however, are hard to interpret. For example, Liew et al. found no identical twins with differences comparable to those seen in Hammond et al.[51] If those specific twins were added to the Liew et al. sample, the heritability coefficient would be dramatically reduced, which raises the question of generalizability. Heritability coefficients, like any other statistic, include error that results from measurement, effect, and sample sizes. As heritability studies go, a sample size of 300 twins is relatively small. Perhaps more importantly, the authors also used an extremely homogenous sample (relatively affluent, young, healthy Caucasian women) with low average MP density. Given the fact that similar environments inflate heritability estimates, the homogeneity of the study sample is an issue. For example, if one were measuring the heritability of height and used all professional basketball players, the estimate would be inflated because most of the differences between all of the tall players would be explainable due to genetic differences. Assuming the measurements are valid,* the most that we can say from the Liew et al. study is that genetic influences can explain a proportion of the differences one is likely to see when measuring young Caucasian women from similar backgrounds.

Secondary Structural Features

A recent question has arisen regarding some of the secondary structural features of MP. As noted, most studies find that the spatial distribution of MP within the human retina is strongly predicted (e.g., usually with $r^2 > 0.90$) as an exponential decline with eccentricity. Hammond et al.,[14] however, originally found that about 40% of their subjects displayed stable deviations from an exponential curve that they described as flanking peaks and valleys. Hammond et al. regarded these secondary spatial perturbations as minor but not artifactual. Recently, however, a number of studies have argued that these spatial deviations can be quite substantial (e.g., Gellermann et al.,[53,54] Berendschot and van Norren,[55] and Delori et al.[56]). There is little doubt that the spatial distribution of MP cannot be described by a perfectly smooth

---

* The overall relation between the AF and HFP measures of MP in the Liew et al. study was low ($r^2 = 0.36$), calling into question whether the measurements were valid. Two methods measuring the same variable in the same subjects should explain more than 36% of the variance.

line. The exact nature and magnitude of these irregularities, however, and how they reflect variations in the architecture of the retina are open to question. For instance, one issue that must be resolved is to what extent these irregularities are real and/or result from noise within the measurements (e.g., see the points raised in Hammond et al.[57]).

THE FUNCTION OF MACULAR PIGMENT

The Protective Hypothesis

Gould and Lewontin[58] originally used the architectural term "spandrel" to describe traits that have evolved yet are nonadaptive. When applied to biology, one can adapt the term to illustrate the point that there are biological traits that serve no purpose and may have simply evolved as "side effects." One must therefore consider the possibility that L and Z actually have no function within the human retina (the null hypothesis). There are, however, many facts that make this possibility unlikely. First, L and Z are very highly concentrated within the fovea, making the fovea the most carotenoid-dense region within the body.[59] In addition, the foveal region of the retina has exaggerated importance in vision. Foveal input is greatly magnified by the striate cortex, and most human visual information processing originates from the sensory input initiated from this small retinal region. If MP served no positive function *in vivo*, it would only serve to reduce the amount of useful light available to this very critical region of the retina. It is probably also not purely incidental that L and Z are antioxidants found within lipid-rich receptoral outer segments (e.g., Rapp et al.[60]), a region that suffers greatly from oxidative damage. It seems, therefore, unlikely that MP is a biological spandrel. Rather, its specific placement and characteristics imply that it serves some important function or functions. Moreover, MP's rather wide variation across individuals implies that whatever functions it serves, MP does not serve these functions equally in all subjects, which begs the question of whether individuals with low MP are at some disadvantage.

Protection and Disease Prevention in the Adult Eye

The idea that MP protects the eye is the idea most widely studied regarding MP's function. Protection of the retina and underlying RPE could be achieved through passive absorption of short-wave light (Figure 5.3). Protection could also be achieved through active quenching of reactive oxygen species that cause damage mostly to lipid membranes (e.g., within photoreceptor outer segments). This antioxidant mechanism could operate in other areas where L and Z are present including the outer layers of the crystalline lens (e.g., Yeum et al.[61]). By preventing actinic and oxidative damage over the life span, L and Z could retard the development of degenerative ocular diseases that result from cumulative damage—namely, age-related cataract (ARC) and age-related macular degeneration (AMD).

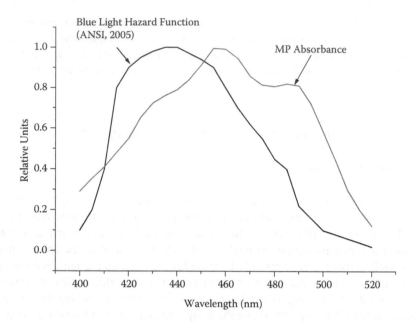

Figure 5.3 The spectral absorbance of macular pigment plotted with the blue light hazard function. (From Hammond, B.R. et al., *Optom. Vis. Sci.*, 82(5), 387–404, 2005.) This function described the potential for photochemical damage to the retina resulting from exposure to light from about 400 to 500 nm as defined by the IESNA Photobiology Committee for ANSI (ANSI/IESNA RP-27.1-05).

Although clearly feasible, the protection hypothesis is difficult to study directly due to the long time course involved. Most of the data available are cross-sectional, inferred from laboratory data, or acute in nature. For example, some researchers have shown that MP is substantially lower in patients with AMD.[62,63] These studies must assume, however, that these subjects always had lower MP levels (i.e., that their current levels accurately reflect their MP levels over the 60–70 years of life preceding the disease) and that some unknown side effect of the disease (e.g., increased oxidative stress) is not lowering or raising MP levels. Such studies are especially difficult to conduct now, given the widespread use of L and Z supplements by AMD patients and the increased availability of such supplements to the general public and high disease risk populations.

Although direct evidence is difficult to obtain, some strong inferences can be made. There is, for instance, abundant evidence that L and Z are highly effective lipid antioxidants (e.g., Sujak et al.[64]). There is even evidence that they serve this function within the retina (e.g., Khachik et al.[65]). It is also clear that the retina suffers from oxidative damage (for review, see Krinsky et al.[36]). Similarly, if it is true that short-wave light in the visible region of the electromagnetic spectrum (400–500 nm) damages the retina (the so-called "blue-light hazard")[66,67] and, since MP attenuates such light (see Figure 5.3), it must also be true that such attenuation is protective. What is less clear is the relative importance of all of these factors. ARC and AMD are clearly multifactorial conditions with complex etiologies. Many lifestyle and genetic factors contribute to the incidence and severity of these diseases. It is extremely difficult to design studies that allow an accurate weighing of all of the relevant factors as they occur over an entire lifetime. For example, short-term studies using high-intensity light have been used to define the blue-light hazard. It is unknown, however, whether these short-term studies, largely on monkeys, are similar enough to the more realistic situation of being exposed to much lower intensities of light for a much longer time period.

Another manifestation of the protective hypothesis does not pertain to protection in its most common connotation (i.e., prevention) per se but, rather, to the idea that supplementing L and Z might actually *treat* some aspects of retinal disease. The retina comprises neural tissue, which, like other central nervous tissue, does not undergo mitosis. Consequently, once damage has been incurred in this region, it is likely that very little can be done to *reverse* that damage, especially when considering advanced stages of the disease process (e.g., blindness in late AMD). *Preventing* degeneration is therefore the most likely benefit that could be expected through L and Z supplementation.

It is possible, however, that supplementing L and Z even late in life or early in the disease process might be beneficial. For example, Mainster[68] recently argued that lipofuscin is a potent photosensitizer* and that its accumulation in retinal tissue creates a cascade, by which lipofuscin accumulation instigates more lipofuscin accumulation. The end result of this cascade is an acceleration of the theoretical point where dysfunction of the retinal pigment epithelium would initiate the disease process. Since the elderly retina has the highest levels of lipofuscin, it may be at highest risk of AMD. Given Mainster's[68] argument that increased lipofuscin accumulation in the elderly retina makes it exceptionally susceptible to blue light damage, L and Z supplementation may be of added benefit in this population (e.g., L and Z have been shown to prevent photo-oxidation of A2-PE/A2E, a major and toxic component of lipofuscin[69]). This possibility becomes especially intriguing given the fact that phototoxicity of lipofuscin (after correction for dense anterior media) well matches the absorption spectrum of MP (peak phototoxicity is approximately 430 nm).[48]

The idea that older retinas may benefit from supplementation of L and Z is not new. Other authors (e.g., Liang and Godley[70] and Wu et al.[71]) have argued that older retinas suffer increased levels of oxidative stress and therefore might benefit from extra antioxidant supplementation. For example, photoreceptor loss (particularly rod loss) is a feature of older retinas and becomes profound in some disease states (e.g., retinitis pigmentosa [RP]). Rod loss can increase oxygen tension, oxygen consumption, and hyperoxia throughout the retina.[72,73] Supplementation with L and Z reduces photoreceptor loss in animal models of RP.[73] In addition, oxidative stress is one possible factor promoting the progression of "dry" AMD to the more severe neovascular

---

* A parallel body of research has identified one of the main fluorophores of lipofuscin, A2E, as particularly toxic to RPE cells (e.g., Sparrow et al.[94]). Evidence indicates that L and Z are protective against A2E photo-oxidation (Kim et al.[69]).

AMD. Indeed, high L and Z intakes are often preferentially associated with reduced rates of the neovascular form of AMD.[74,75]

Protection by MP of the Infant Retina

Bone et al.[20] originally showed that MP was as highly variable in the infant retina as it is in the adult retina. Z is the dominant carotenoid in the center of the adult retina and L predominates in the periphery (thus, *in vivo* measures of MP account mostly for zeaxanthin concentration). This ratio appears to be reversed in the infant retina, where L dominates in the center (at this point, of course, the macula is quite immature and similar to the periphery). Although all of the factors responsible for the wide variation in infant MP have not been studied, dietary intake of L and Z is still clearly necessary. Whereas MP can be manipulated in the adult via intake of xanthophyll-rich foods, the obvious concern with infants is that food options are limited to breast milk or manufactured infant formulas. Breast milk contains at least 300 defined nutrients, whereas most infant formulas contain approximately 60–70 defined nutrients.[76] Currently, infant formula does not contain L and Z in other than trace amounts,[76] and many formulas are completely devoid of L. In contrast, breast milk contains L and Z in concentrations that are approximately proportional to maternal intake of these carotenoids.[77] These observations are important since many infants are exclusively formula fed. Johnson et al.[21] showed that breast-fed infants and formula-fed infants had the same levels of plasma L and Z at birth. After 1 month, however, plasma L and Z significantly increased for the breast-fed infants and decreased in the formula-fed infants. This implies that retinal levels in formula-fed infants are also low.

We do not know what the effects are of the relative absence of L and Z (i.e., in formula-fed infants or in breast-fed infants with mothers with low dietary intake of L and Z) on the rapidly developing and still immature macula (see the review by Zimmer and Hammond[78]). The effects, however, are probably not positive.* The adult retina is a tissue that is at high risk of oxidation. All of the elements necessary for oxidative damage are present in abundance in the adult retina, such as high lipid content, oxygen tension, and photosensitizers (e.g., A2E). These conditions are also present in the infant retina. Moreover, the crystalline lens of the infant transmits a higher percentage of damaging short-wave light than the adult retina.[79] A recent study of children in Australia[80] showed that fully one-third of children tested had increased fluorescence of the sclera (thickened conjunctiva, called pinguecula), indicating clinically significant ocular damage from the sun. This may be one reason why lipofuscin (largely oxidized lipids accumulating as debris mostly within the RPE) accumulation is so rapid in young children[81,82] (see Figure 5.4.).

---

* It is possible that absence of L and Z during infancy and childhood cause architectural changes in the retina and underlying RPE. Leung et al.[95] have recently shown that monkeys raised on chow deficient in L and Z and omega fatty acids showed substantial anatomical changes in their RPE compared to monkeys raised with normal chow.

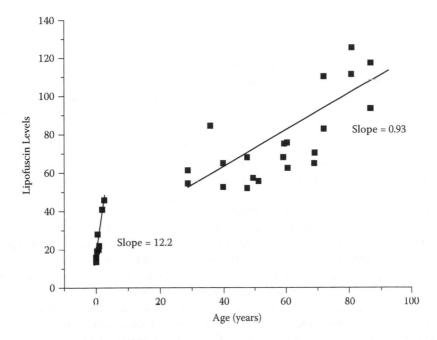

Figure 5.4 The levels of the autofluorescence pigment lipofuscin as a function of age. Lipofuscin accumulates within the retinal pigment epithelium as a result of oxidative damage to lipid membranes within the retina and is often regarded as a marker of the health of the retinal/RPE complex. (Data derived from Wing, G.L. et al., *Invest. Ophthalmol. Vis. Sci.*, 17(7), 601–607, 1978.)

Optical Hypotheses

The previously mentioned hypotheses suggest that MP is capable of preventing disease by influencing biological processes of the retina. Another possibility is that supplementation by L and Z, even if they have no impact on the biology of the disease, could treat the symptoms (i.e., visual loss) of disease. This possibility is based on the idea that MP could improve visual performance through optical mechanisms.

The idea that yellow filters could improve visual performance has a long history. The idea was well summarized by Walls and Judd,[83] who argued that the ubiquity of intraocular yellow filters in nature (as opposed to retinal filters with other absorptive qualities, such as red filters) was evidence for the idea that yellow filters play an important role in vision. One common manifestation of this idea is the use of yellow goggles to improve visual performance outdoors (see the discussion by Wooten and Hammond[84]). Following Walls and Judd's initial presentation of this argument, Nussbaum et al.[85] later suggested that MP, the intraocular yellow filter of humans, could serve the functions originally outlined by Walls and Judd:

1. To increase visual acuity by reducing chromatic aberration
2. To promote comfort by the reduction of glare and dazzle

3. To enhance detail by the absorption of "blue haze"
4. To enhance contrast

The first of these four functions outlined by Walls and Judd, commonly referred to as the acuity hypothesis, is widely stated in the literature as fact but has only recently been empirically tested. The acuity hypothesis is based on the well-known properties of chromatic aberration (CA). Any time visible light is refracted by a lens made of a single refractive material, the light will be focused at different planes, depending on wavelength. For instance, when one is viewing a broadband (whitish) light, only the middle wavelengths (greenish-yellow light) are focused on the retina (these wavelengths often serve as the accommodation signal). The shorter wavelengths (bluish light) are focused considerably far in front of the retina (more than 1.5 diopters) and the longer wavelengths (reddish light) are focused behind the retina. Theoretically, out-of-focus blue light would blur the edges of an image and reduce acuity proportionally. By absorbing the out-of-focus light, MP could sharpen an image and increase acuity (e.g., see the model by Reading and Weale[86]).

Although feasible, the acuity hypothesis has several problems. First, it applies only to broadband light because the young lens can accommodate to stimuli viewed under narrowband conditions. Second, there is the possibility that the eye suffers from so many optical distortions that any theoretical reduction by CA is simply washed out by the many other sources of distortion.[87] Recently, Engles et al.[89] tested the acuity hypothesis by measuring hyperacuity and gap acuity in broadband light, which is absorbed by MP, and yellowish light, which is not absorbed by MP. Engles et al. found that MP did not improve acuity in either condition. These data strongly suggest that MP does not improve acuity by reducing the effects of CA.

The second of the four previously mentioned functions, known as the glare hypothesis, is based on the idea that MP could reduce the discomfort and disability caused by viewing objects under glare conditions. As a filter, MP would certainly reduce some of the intraocular scatter associated with a glaring light source. The question is whether filtering essentially only about a third of the visible spectrum (i.e., the shortwave end) is sufficient to reduce discomfort and disability. This question was tested by Stringham et al.[88,90] Stringham et al.[88] characterized visual discomfort using electromyogram (EMG) recordings of the squint response. From this they generated a photophobia (acute glare discomfort) action spectrum, which peaked at 460 nm. Stringham et al., in fact, showed that MP reduced photophobia in a direct linear fashion. More recently, Stringham et al.[90] have shown that MP increases the visibility of a target when veiled by a glare source. This effect was quite strong (correlation values of about 0.7–0.8).

The final function is based on the idea that any time MP absorbs a surround or background more than a target (or vice versa) contrast will be enhanced and vision will improve. This kind of contrast enhancement easily translates to vision outdoors, where MP could improve vision by absorbing blue haze or skylight (in this application, termed the visibility hypothesis[84]) more than objects seen against those backgrounds. Such "targets" often have longer wavelengths than their background since Rayleigh scatter would tend to redden distant objects viewed along the sightline. Although the visibility hypothesis is clearly feasible and has been extensively modeled,[84] there are currently no empirical data available to evaluate the validity of the hypothesis.

All of the preceding represent optical means by which MP could improve vision. MP could also improve visual function, however, simply by promoting a healthier retina. Richer et al.,[91] for example, using a double-masked, placebo-controlled, randomized trial study design, supplemented AMD subjects (elderly veterans) and controls with 10 mg of L or alone or with a mixed antioxidant supplement and found increased MP density, increased contrast sensitivity, decreased glare disability, and increased Snellen acuity compared to matched controls. A similar result, obtained using a similarly rigorous experimental design, was obtained on cataract subjects by Olmedilla et al.[92]

CONCLUSION

MP is a major component of the fovea. It is likely that MP serves both to protect the retina and to improve some aspects of visual performance (such as vision under glare conditions). All other things being equal, individuals with low levels of MP (such as formula-fed infants, adults with low dietary intakes of xanthophyll-rich foods, and individuals with certain retinal diseases) are probably at a disadvantage compared to individuals with high levels of MP. Supplementation with purified lutein and/or zeaxanthin esters can increase MP density in most individuals, as can supplementation via carotenoid-rich whole foods. The effects of increasing MP density on retinal health across the life span is unknown but is generally thought to be significant.

REFERENCES

1. Wald, G. Human vision and the spectrum, *Nature*, 101, 653–658, 1945.
2. Bone, R.A., Landrum, J.T., and Tarsis, S.L. Preliminary identification of the human macular pigment, *Vision Res.*, 25, 1531–1539, 1985.
3. Bone, R.A., Landrum, J.T., Hime, G.W., Cains, A., and Zamor, J. Stereochemistry of the human macular carotenoids, *Invest. Ophthalmol. Vis. Sci.*, 34(6), 2033–2040, 1993.
4. Khachik, F., Moura, F.F., Zhao, D.Y., Aebischer, C.P., and Bernstein, P.S. Transformations of selected carotenoids in plasma, liver and ocular tissues of humans and in nonprimate animal models, *Invest. Ophthalmol. Vis. Sci.*, 43, 3383–3392, 2002.
5. Johnson, E.J., Neuringer, M., Russell, R.M., Schalch, W., and Snodderly, D.M. Nutritional manipulation of primate retinas. III. Effects of lutein or zeaxanthin supplementation on adipose tissue and retina of xanthophyll-free monkeys, *Invest. Ophthalmol. Vis. Sci.*, 46(2), 692–702, 2005.
6. Mares-Perlman, J.A., Millen, A.E., Ficek, T.L., and Hankinson, S.E. The body of evidence to support a protective role for lutein and zeaxanthin in delaying chronic disease. Overview, *J. Nutr.*, 132, 518S–524S, 2002.
7. Parker, R.S. Absorption, metabolism and transport of carotenoids, *FASEB J.*, 10, 542–551, 1996.

8. Clevidence, B.A., and Bieri, J.G. Association of carotenoids with human plasma lipo-proteins, *Methods Enzymol.*, 214, 33–46, 1993.
9. Bernstein, P.S., Balashov, N.A., Tsong, E.D., and Rando, R.R. Retinal tubulin binds macular carotenoids, *Invest. Ophthalmol. Vis. Sci.*, 38, 167–175, 1997.
10. Yemelyanov, A.Y., Katz, N.B., and Bernstein, P.S. Ligand-binding characterization of xan-thophyll carotenoids to solubilized membrane proteins derived from human retina, *Exp. Eye Res.*, 72, 381–392, 2001.
11. Crabtree, D.V., Ojima, I., Geng, X., and Adler, A.J. Tubulins in the primate retina: Evidence that xanthophylls may be endogenous ligands for the paclitaxel-binding site, *Bioorg. Med. Chem.*, 9, 1967–1976, 2001.
12. Bhosale, P., Larson, A.J., Frederick, J.M., Southwick, K., Thulin, C.D., and Bernstein, P.S. Identification and characterization of a Pi isoform of glutathione S-transferase ($GSTP_1$) as a zeaxanthin-binding protein in the macula of the human eye, *J. Biol. Chem.*, 279(47), 49447–49454, 2004.
13. Snodderly, D.M., Handelman, G.J., and Adler, A.J. Distribution of individual macular pig-ment carotenoids in central retina of macaque and squirrel monkeys, *Invest. Ophthalmol. Vis. Sci.*, 32, 268–279, 1991.
14. Hammond, B.R., Johnson, E.J., Russell, R.M., Krinsky, N.I., Yeum, K.J., Edwards, R.B., and Snodderly, D.M. Individual variations in the spatial profile of macular pigment, *J. Am. Optom. Assoc.*, 14(6), 1187–1196, 1997.
15. Wooten, B.R., and Hammond, B.R. Spectral absorbance and spatial distribution of macu-lar pigment using heterochromatic flicker photometry, *Optom. Vis. Sci.*, 82(5), 378–386, 2005.
16. Bernstein, P.S., Khachik, F., Carvalho, L.S., Muir, G.J., Zhao, D.-Y., and Katz, N.B. Identi-fication and quantification of carotenoids and their metabolites in the tissues of the human eye, *Exp. Eye Res.*, 72, 215–223, 2001.
17. Craft, N.E., Haitema, H.B., Garnett, K.M., Fitch, K.A., and Dorey, C.K. Carotenoid, tocoph-erol and retinol concentrations in the elderly human brain, *J. Nutr. Health Aging*, 8(3), 156–162, 2004.
18. Ciulla, T.A., Curran-Celentano, J., Cooper, D.A., Hammond, B.R., Danis, R.P., Pratt, L.M. et al. Macular pigment optical density in a Midwestern sample, *Ophthalmology*,108, 730–737, 2001.
19. Hammond, B.R., and Caruso-Avery, M. Macular pigment optical density in a Southwestern sample, *Invest. Ophthalmol. Vis. Sci.*, 41(6), 1492–1497, 2000.
20. Bone, R.A., Landrum, J.T., Fernandez, L., and Tarsis, S.L. Analysis of the macular pig-ment by HPLC: Retinal distribution and age study, *Invest. Ophthalmol. Vis. Sci.*, 29(6), 843–849, 1988.
21. Johnson, L., Norkus, E., Abbasi, S., Gerdes, J.S., and Bhutani, V.K. Contribution of beta-carotene (BC) from BC-enriched formulae to individual and total serum carotenoids in term infants, *FASEB J.*, 9(4 Pt 3): Abstract no. 1869, 1995.
22. Hibino, H. Red-green and yellow-blue opponent-color responses as a function of retinal eccentricity, *Vision Res.*, 32(10), 1955–1964, 1992.
23. Stringham, J., and Hammond, B.R. Compensation for macular pigment: Relation to hue-cancellation thresholds, *Ophthalmol. Physio. Opt.*, 27, 232–237, 2007.
24. Wooten, B.R., Hammond, B.R., Land, R.I., and Snodderly, D.M. A practical method for mea-suring macular pigment optical density, *Invest. Ophthalmol. Vis. Sci.*, 40(11), 2481–2489, 1999.
25. Delori, F.C. Autofluorescence method to measure macular pigment optical densities fluo-rometry and autofluorescence imaging, *Arch. Biochem. Biophys.*, 430(2), 156–162, 2004.

26. Berendschot, T.T.J.M., and van Norren, D. Objective determination of the macular pigment optical density using fundus reflectance spectroscopy, *Arch. Biochem. Biophys.*, 430(2), 149–155, 2004.

27. Gellermann, W., Ermakov, I.V., Ermakova, M.R., McClane, R.W., Wintch, S.W., Zhao, D.Y., and Bernstein, P.S. Raman detection of carotenoid pigments in the human retina, *Proc. SPIE*, 4245, 146–157, 2001.

28. Hammond, B.R., Wooten, B.R., and Smollon, B. Assessment of the validity of *in vivo* methods of measuring human macular pigment optical density, *Optom. Vis. Sci.*, 82(5), 387–404, 2005.

29. Neelam, K., O'Gorman, N., Nolan, J., O'Donovan, O., Wong, H.B., Au Eong, K.G. et al. Measurement of macular pigment: Raman spectroscopy vs. heterochromatic flicker photometry, *Invest. Ophthalmol. Vis. Sci.*, 46(3), 1023–1032, 2005.

30. Sharifzadeh, M., Bernstein, P.S., and Gellermann, W. Nonmydriatic fluorescence-based quantitative imaging of human macular pigment distributions, *J. Opt. Soc. Am. A.*, 23(10), 2373–2387, 2006.

31. Hammond, B.R., and Wooten, B.R. Resonance Raman spectroscopic measurement of carotenoids in the skin and retina, *J. Biomed. Opt.*, 10(5), 054002, 2005.

32. Delori, F.C., Goger, D.G., Hammond, B.R., Snodderly, D.M., and Burns, S.A. Macular pigment density measured by autofluorescence spectrometry: Comparison with reflectometry and heterochromatic flicker photometry, *J. Opt. Soc. Am. A.*, 18(6), 1212–1230, 2001.

33. Curran-Celentano, J., Hammond, B.R., Ciulla, T.A., Cooper, D.A., Pratt, L.M., and Danis, R.B. Relation between dietary intake, serum concentrations and retinal concentrations of lutein and zeaxanthin in adults in a Midwest population, *Am. J. Clin. Nutr.*, 74, 796–802, 2001.

34. Hammond, B.R., Curran-Celentano, J., Judd, S., Fuld, K., Krinsky, N.I., Wooten, B.R., and Snodderly, D.M. Sex differences in macular pigment optical density: Relation to plasma carotenoid concentrations and dietary patterns, *Vision Res.*, 36(13), 2001–2012, 1996.

35. Hammond, B.R., Johnson, E.J., Russell, R.M., Krinsky, N.I., Yeum, K.J., Edwards, R.B., and Snodderly, D.M. Dietary modification of human macular pigment density, *Invest. Ophthalmol. Vis. Sci.*, 38(9), 1795–1801, 1997.

36. Krinsky, N.I., Landrum, J.T., and Bone, R.A. Biologic mechanisms of the protective role of lutein and zeaxanthin in the eye, *Annu. Rev. Nutr.*, 23, 171–201, 2003.

37. Beatty, S., Nolan, J., Kavanagh, H., and O'Donovan, O. Macular pigment optical density and its relationship with serum and dietary levels of lutein and zeaxanthin, *Arch. Biochem. Biophys.*, 430, 70–76, 2004.

38. Schupp, C., Olano-Martin, E., Gerth, C., Morrissey, B.M., Cross, C.E., and Werner, J.S. Lutein, zeaxanthin, macular pigment and visual function in adult cystic fibrosis patients, *Am. J. Clin. Nutr.*, 79(6), 1045–1052, 2004.

39. Davies, N.P., and Morland, A.B. Color matching in diabetes: Optical density of the crystalline lens and macular pigments, *Invest. Ophthalmol. Vis. Sci.*, 43, 281–289, 2002.

40. Zagers, N.P., Pot, M.C., and van Norren, D. Spectral and directional reflectance of the fovea in diabetes mellitus: Photoreceptor integrity, macular pigment and lens, *Vision Res.*, 45(13), 1745–1753, 2005.

41. Aleman, T.S., Duncan, J.L., Bieber, M.L., de Castro, E., Marks, D.A., Gardner, L.M. et al. Macular pigment and lutein supplementation in retinitis pigmentosa and Usher syndrome, *Invest. Ophthalmol. Vis. Sci.*, 42(8), 1873–1881, 2001.

42. Duncan, J.L., Aleman, T.S., Gardner, L.M., de Castro, E., Marks, D.A., Emmons, J.M. et al. Macular pigment and lutein supplementation in choroideremia, *Exp. Eye Res.*, 74(3), 371–381, 2002.

43. Whitehead, A.J., Mares, J.A., and Danis, R.P. Macular pigment: A review of current knowledge, *Arch. Ophthalmol.*, 124(7), 1038–1045, 2006.
44. Gellermann, W., Ermakov, I.V., Ermakova, M.R., McClane, R.W., Zhao, D.Y., and Bernstein, P.S. In vivo resonant Raman measurement of macular carotenoid pigments in the young and the aging human retina, *J. Opt. Soc. Am. A.*, 19(6), 1172–1186, 2002.
45. Nolan, J.M., Stack, J., O'Donovan, O., Loane, E., and Beatty, S. Risk factors for age-related maculopathy are associated with a relative lack of macular pigment, *Exp. Eye Res.*, 84, 61–74, 2007.
46. Beatty, S., Murray, I.J., Henson, D.B., Carden, D., Koh, H., and Boulton, M.E. Macular pigment and risk for age-related macular degeneration in subjects from a Northern European population, *Invest. Ophthalmol. Vis. Sci.*, 42(2), 439–446, 2001.
47. Ciulla, T.A., and Hammond, B.R. Macular pigment density and aging, assessed in the normal elderly and those with cataracts and age-related macular degeneration, *Am. J. Ophthalmol.*, 138(4), 582–587, 2004.
48. Berendschot, T.T.J.M., and van Norren, D. On age dependency of the macular pigment optical density, *Exp. Eye Res.*, 81(5), 602–609, 2005.
49. Hammond, B.R., and Johnson, M.A. Dietary prevention and treatment of age-related macular degeneration, *Recent Res. Devel. Nutrition*, 5, 43–68, 2002.
50. Handelman, G.J., Snodderly, D.M., Krinsky, N.I., Russett, M.D., and Adler, A.J. Biological control of primate macular pigment. Biochemical and densitometric studies, *Invest. Ophthalmol. Vis. Sci.*, 32(2), 257–267, 1991.
51. Hammond, B.R., Fuld, K., and Curran-Celentano, J. Macular pigment density in monozygotic twins, *Invest. Ophthalmol. Vis. Sci.*, 36(12), 2531–2541, 1995.
52. Liew, S.H., Gilbert, C.E., Spector, T.D., Mellerio, J., Marshall, J., van Kuijk, F. et al. Heritability of macular pigment: A twin study, *Invest. Ophthalmol. Vis. Sci.*, 46(12), 4430–4436, 2005.
53. Gellermann, W. Ermakov, I.V., McClane, R.W., and Bernstein, P.S. Raman imaging of human macular pigments, *Opt. Lett.*, 27, 833–835, 2002.
54. Gellermann, W., Ermakov, I.V., and McClane, R.W. Raman imaging of carotenoid pigments in human retina, *Proc. SPIE*, 4611, 197–207, 2002.
55. Berendschot, T.T.J.M., and van Norren, D. Macular pigment shows ringlike structures, *Invest. Ophthalm. Vis. Sci.*, 47(2), 709–714, 2006.
56. Delori, F.C., Goger, D.G., Keilhauer, C., Salvetti, P., and Staurenghi, G. Bimodal spatial distribution of macular pigment: Evidence of a gender relationship, *J. Opt. Soc. Am. A.*, 23(3), 521–538, 2006.
57. Hammond, B.R., Wooten, B.R., and Smollon, B. Response to Gellermann, W., and Bernstein, P.S., *Optom. Vis. Sci.*, 83(4), 254–259, 2006.
58. Gould, S.J., and Lewontin, R.C. The spandrels of San Marco and the Panglossian paradigm: A critique of the adaptationist program, *Proc. R. Soc. Lond. B.*, 205, 581–598, 1979.
59. Landrum, J.T., Bone, R.A., Moore, L.L., and Gomez, C.M. Analysis of zeaxanthin distribution within individual human retinas, *Methods Enzymol.*, 299, 457–467, 1999.
60. Rapp, L.M., Maple, S.S., and Choi, J.H. Lutein and zeaxanthin concentrations in rod outer segment membranes from perifoveal and peripheral human retina, *Invest. Ophthalmol. Vis. Sci.*, 41(5), 1200–1209, 2000.
61. Yeum, K.J., Taylor, A., Tang, G., and Russell, R.M. Measurement of carotenoids, retinoids and tocopherols in human lenses, *Invest. Ophthalmol. Vis. Sci.*, 36(13), 2756–2761, 1995.
62. Bone, R.A., Landrum, J.T., Mayne, S.T., Gomez, C.M., Tibor, S.E., and Twaroska, E.E. Macular pigment in donor eyes with and without AMD: A case-control study, *Invest. Ophthalmol. Vis. Sci.*, 42(1), 235–240, 2001.

63. Beatty, S., Murray, I.J., Henson, D.B., Carden, D., Koh, H., and Boulton, M.E. Macular pigment and risk for age-related macular degeneration in subjects from a Northern European population, *Invest. Ophthalmol. Vis. Sci.*, 42(2), 439–446, 2001.

64. Sujak, A., Gabrielska, J. Grudzinski, W., Borc, R., Mazurek, P., and Gruszecki, W.I. Lutein and zeaxanthin as protectors of lipid membranes against oxidative damage: The structural aspects, *Arch. Biochem. Biophys.*, 371, 301–307, 1999.

65. Khachik, F., Bernstein, P.S., and Garland, D.L. Identification of lutein and zeaxanthin oxidation products in human and monkey retinas, *Invest. Ophthalmol. Vis. Sci.*, 38(9), 1802–1811, 1997.

66. Ham, W.T., Ruffolo, J.J., Mueller, H.A., Clarke, A.M., and Moon, M.E. Histologic analysis of photochemical lesions produced in rhesus retina by short wave-length light, *Invest. Ophthalmol. Vis. Sci.*, 17, 1029–1035, 1978.

67. van Norren, D., and Schellekens, P. Blue light hazard in rat, *Vision Res.*, 30(10), 1517–1520, 1990.

68. Mainster, M.A. Violet and blue light blocking intraocular lenses: Photoprotection versus photoreception, *Br. J. Ophthalmol.*, 90(6), 784–792, 2006.

69. Kim, S.R., Nakanishi, K., Itagaki, Y., and Sparrow, J.R. Photooxidation of A2-PE, a photoreceptor outer segment fluorophore, and protection by lutein and zeaxanthin, *Exp. Eye Res.*, 82(5), 828–839, 2006.

70. Liang, F.Q., and Godley, B.F. Oxidative stress-induced mitochondrial DNA damage in human retinal pigment epithelial cells: A possible mechanism for RPE aging and age-related macular degeneration, *Exp. Eye Res.*, 76, 397–403, 2003.

71. Wu, J., Seregard, S., and Algvere, P.V. Photochemical damage of the retina, *Surv. Ophthalmol.*, 51(5), 461–481, 2006.

72. Shen, J., Yang, X., Dong, A., Petters, R., Peng, Y-W., Wong, F. et al. Oxidative damage is a potential cause of cone cell death in retinitis pigmentosa, *J. Cell. Physiol.*, 203, 457–464, 2005.

73. Komeima, K., Rogers, B.S., Lu, L., and Campochiaro, P.A. Antioxidants reduce cone cell death in a model of retinitis pigmentosa, *PNAS*, 103(30), 11300–11305, 2006.

74. Eye Disease Case-Control Study Group. Risk factors for neovascular age-related macular degeneration, *Arch. Ophthalmol.*, 110, 1701–1708, 1992.

75. Eye Disease Case-Control Study Group. Antioxidant status and neovascular age-related macular degeneration, *Arch. Ophthalmol.*, 111, 104–109, 1993.

76. Jewell, V.C., Mayes C.B.D., Tubman, T.R.J., Northrop-Clewes, C.A., and Thurnham, D.I. A comparison of lutein and zeaxanthin concentrations in formula and human milk samples from Northern Ireland mothers, *Eur. J. Clin. Nutr.*, 58, 90–97, 2004.

77. Jewell, V.C., Sweet, D., Tubman, T.R.J., Northrop-Clewes, C.A., and Thurnham, D.I. Lutein and zeaxanthin levels in newborn infants and their mothers, *Proc. Nutr. Soc.*, 59, 47A, 2000.

78. Zimmer, P., and Hammond, B.R.. Lutein and zeaxanthin and the developing retina, *Clin. Ophthalmol.*, 1, 181–189, 2007.

79. Dillon, J., Zheng, L., Merriam, J.C., and Gaillard, E.R. Transmission of light to the aging human retina: Possible implications for age-related macular degeneration, *Exp. Eye Res.*, 79(6), 753–759, 2004.

80. Ooi, J.L., Sharma, N.S., Papalkar, D., Sharma, S., Oakey, M., Dawes, P. et al. Ultraviolet fluorescence photography to detect early sun damage in the eyes of school-aged children, *Am. J. Ophthalmol.*, 141(2), 294–298, 2006.

81. Wing, G.L., Blanchard, G.C., and Weiter, J.J. The topography and age relationship of lipo-fuscin concentration in the retinal pigment epithelium, *Invest. Ophthalmol. Vis. Sci.*, 17(7), 601–607, 1978.

82. Feeney-Burns, L., Hilderbrand, E.S., and Eldridge, S. Aging human RPE: Morphometric analysis of macular, equatorial, and peripheral cells, *Invest. Ophthalmol. Vis. Sci.*, 25(2), 195–200, 1984.

83. Walls, G.L., and Judd, H.D. Intra-ocular color filters of vertebrates, *Br. J. Ophthalmol.*, 17, 641–725, 1933.

84. Wooten, B.R., and Hammond, B.R. Macular pigment: Influences on visual acuity and vis-ibility, *Prog. Retinal Eye Res.*, 21, 225–240, 2002.

85. Nussbaum, J.J., Pruett, R.C., and Delori, F.C. Historic perspectives. Macular yellow pig-ment. The first 200 years, *Retina*, 1(4), 296–310, 1981.

86. Reading, V.M., and Weale, R.A. Macular pigment and chromatic aberration, *J. Am. Optom. Assoc.*, 64(2), 231–234, 1974.

87. McLellan, J.S., Marcos, S., Prieto, P.M., and Burns, S.A. Imperfect optics may be the eye's defense against chromatic blur, *Nature*, 417, 174–176, 2002.

88. Stringham, J.M., Fuld, K., and Wenzel, A.J. Action spectrum for photophobia, *J.Opt. Soc. Am. A*, 20, 1852–1858, 2003.

89. Engles, M., Hammond, B.R., and Wooten, B.R. The relation between macular pigment and resolution acuity. *Invest. Ophthalmol. Vis. Sci.,* 48, 2922–2931, 2007.

90. Stringham, J.M., and Hammond, B.R. The glare hypothesis of macular pigment function. *Opt. Vis. Sci.*, 84(9), 859–864, 2007.

91. Richer, S., Stiles, W., Statkute, L., Pulido, J., Frankowski, J., Rudy, D. et al. Double-masked, placebo-controlled, randomized trial of lutein and antioxidant supplementation in the inter-vention of atrophic age-related macular degeneration: The Veterans LAST Study (lutein antioxidant supplementation trial), *Optometry*, 75(4), 216–230, 2004.

92. Olmedilla, B., Granado, F., Blanco, I. et al. Lutein, but not alpha-tocopherol, supplemen-tation improves visual function in patients with age-related cataracts: A 2-y double-blind, placebo-controlled pilot study, *Nutrition*, 19(1), 21–24, 2003.

93. Malinow, M.R. et al. Diet-related macular anomalies in monkeys, *Invest. Ophthalmol. Vis. Sci.*, 19(8), 857–863, 1980.

94. Sparrow, J.R. et al. The lipofuscin fluorophore A2E mediates blue-light induced damage to retinal pigment epithelial cells, *Invest. Ophthalmol. Vis. Sci.*, 41, 1981–1989, 2000.

95. Leung, I.Y-F. et al. Nutritional manipulation of primate retinas. II. Effects of age, n-3 fatty acids, lutein and zeaxanthin on retinal pigment epithelium, *Invest. Ophthalmol. Vis. Sci.*, 45(9), 3244–3256, 2006.

CHAPTER 6

Phytochemicals and the Aging Brain

Stéphane Bastianetto and Rémi Quirion

CONTENTS

INTRODUCTION

Alzheimer's disease (AD) is one of the most common forms of dementia that affect the elderly population. The histopathological hallmarks of AD are extracellular deposits known as neuritic amyloid plaques and intraneuronal inclusions composed of hyperphosphorylated tangles enriched with tau proteins.[1] The principal component of the neuritic plaques is aggregation of amyloid (Aβ), which is likely to play a role in the neurodegenerative process. The relative contribution of the various forms (soluble dimers, small oligomers, protofibrils, and fibrils) of Aβ to neuronal dysfunction in neurodegenerative diseases is still debatable.[2,3] Hence, it has been postulated that the progressive accumulation of large intracellular and extracellular Aβ aggregates is not fundamental to the initial development of neurodegenerative pathology that contributes to the progression of AD.[2] Indeed, there is a weak correlation between fibrillar Aβ load and neurological dysfunctions observed in AD. Moreover, Aβ deposits may also develop in cognitively normal individuals who have no evidence of local neuron damage.[2]

On the other hand, recent findings indicate that soluble Aβ oligomers may represent the primary pathologic species in these diseases.[3] Preliminary analyses have revealed abundant soluble oligomers in AD patients, consistent with the idea that oligomers precede senile plaque development and may be linked to cognitive impairments.[3] To date, available drugs for the treatment of AD are somewhat beneficial but cannot markedly reduce the progression of the disease. Therefore, based on these observations, it has been suggested that inhibition of Aβ aggregation may be an appropriate strategy to block or even reverse the progression of the disease.

Epidemiological studies have shown that consumption of fruits, vegetables, green tea, and red wine (in moderation) reduces the incidence of developing neurodegenerative diseases, including Alzheimer's disease.[4–8] Polyphenols that are abundant in these foods and beverages likely contribute to their beneficial effects. In support of this hypothesis, a 5-year follow-up study demonstrated an inverse correlation between flavonoid intake and the risk of dementia.[9] Moreover, *in vitro* and *in vivo* studies have reported that polyphenolic constituents (e.g., resveratrol, catechins, flavonols) protected neurons from Aβ toxicity.[10–15] Finally, a standardized ginkgo biloba extract, a well-known polyphenols-derived natural extract that is prescribed in many countries for the treatment of Alzheimer's disease and cognitive disorders,[16] protected cells from Aβ toxicity[17,18] and alleviated deficits of spatial memory in 14-month-old transgenic mice (Tg2576) that develop Aβ plaques.[19]

Different hypotheses have been raised to explain these purported beneficial effects. Ono et al. have shown that the neuroprotective effects of various polyphenols (e.g., myricetin, morin, and, to a lesser extent, quercetin) may be due to their ability to inhibit amyloid fibrils and to destabilize fibrilized forms of Aβ,[20] suggesting that they could be considered as new therapeutic agents for the treatment of Aβ-associated diseases.[21] Resveratrol, a red-wine polyphenol, has been proposed to promote the intracellular degradation of Aβ by a proteasome-dependent and secretase-independent activity.[22] Based on these findings, we compared the effects of polyphenols found in teas and red wine, using the model of Aβ-induced toxicity in rat hippocampal primary cell cultures.

MATERIALS AND METHODS

Mixed Hippocampal Cell Cultures

Hippocampal cell cultures were prepared from E19 fetuses obtained from Sprague–Dawley rats. Animal care was according to protocols and guidelines of the

McGill University Animal Care Committee and the Canadian Council for Animal Care. Mixed (glial/neuronal) hippocampal cells were obtained as described in detail elsewhere.[10,11]

Experimental Treatments

Aβ-induced toxicity and measurement of cell survival/injury were performed as described in detail elsewhere.[10,11] Briefly, 6-day-old cells were exposed to fresh solutions of either $A\beta_{25-35}$ or $A\beta_{1-42}$ for 24 h, in the presence or absence of different drugs. Cell survival and extent of cell death were determined using MTT and Sytox® green assays, respectively. Measurement of intracellular reactive oxygen species was determined by dichlorofluorescein (DCF) fluorescence assay, as described previously.[23]

Measurement of Soluble and Insoluble (Aggregated) Forms of Aβ

4,4'-Dianilino-1,1'-binaphthyl-5,5'-disulfonate (bis-ANS) is a probe that has been shown to increase in fluorescence with soluble Aβ in acidic buffer solutions.[24] Briefly, $A\beta_{1-42}$ was incubated for 30 minutes at room temperature in the presence of different polyphenols. Bis-ANS fluorescence (excitation = 360 nm, emission = 485 nm) was then measured by dilution of 100-μl aliquots in a final volume of 300 μl of citrate buffer (30 mM, pH 2.4) containing bis-ANS (25 μM), using a fluorescence multiwell plate reader (Bio-Tek Instruments®, Inc.). To determine amyloid fibril formation, the thioflavin T (Th-T) fluorescence method was performed as previously described.[24] Briefly, a fresh solution of $A\beta_{1-42}$ was incubated at 37°C for 24 hours in phosphate-buffered saline (pH 7.4). After incubation, a 100-μl aliquot of solution was added in a final volume of 300 μl of phosphate buffer (50 mM, pH 6.0) containing 5 μM Th-T in the presence of different drugs. Fluorescence was then monitored at excitation and emission wavelengths of 450 and 485 nm, respectively.

RESULTS

Neuroprotective Effect of Resveratrol against Aβ-Induced Neurotoxicity

As expected, application of Aβ peptides ($A\beta_{25-35}$, 20 μM; $A\beta_{1-42}$, 15–20 μM) caused about 40% cell death that was dose-dependently reduced in the presence of pre- and co-treatments of resveratrol (15–40 μM), with a maximal effect obtained at 25 μM. A pretreatment with the protein kinase C (PKC) inhibitor GF 109203X (1 μM) significantly reduced the neuroprotective effects of resveratrol against $A\beta_{25-35}$-induced cytotoxicity. In contrast, inhibitors of MAP kinase (PD98059, 25 μM) and PI3 kinase (LY294002, 5 μM) failed to modulate the neuroprotective action of resveratrol. Based on the role of phosphorylation of PKC in cell survival,[15] we next investigated if resveratrol was able to promote phosphorylation. Western blot suggested that resveratrol (20–30 μM) induced phosphorylation of PKC and abolished the inhibitory effect of $A\beta_{25-35}$ on phosphorylation of PKC as well, thus supporting the role of PKC in the neuroprotective action of resveratrol.

Effects of Tea Extracts and Related Polyphenols against Toxicity Induced by Aβ Peptides

The neurotoxic effect of $A\beta_{25-35}$ was reduced, in a dose-dependent manner by a treatment with green tea extract. These effects are significant at 5 μg/ml and maximal at the highest dose tested here (25 μg/ml). Similarly, the black tea extract that contains 80% of theaflavins (condensed products of catechins; Figure 6.1) appeared to be even more potent and completely protected cells at 5 μg/ml. The neuroprotective

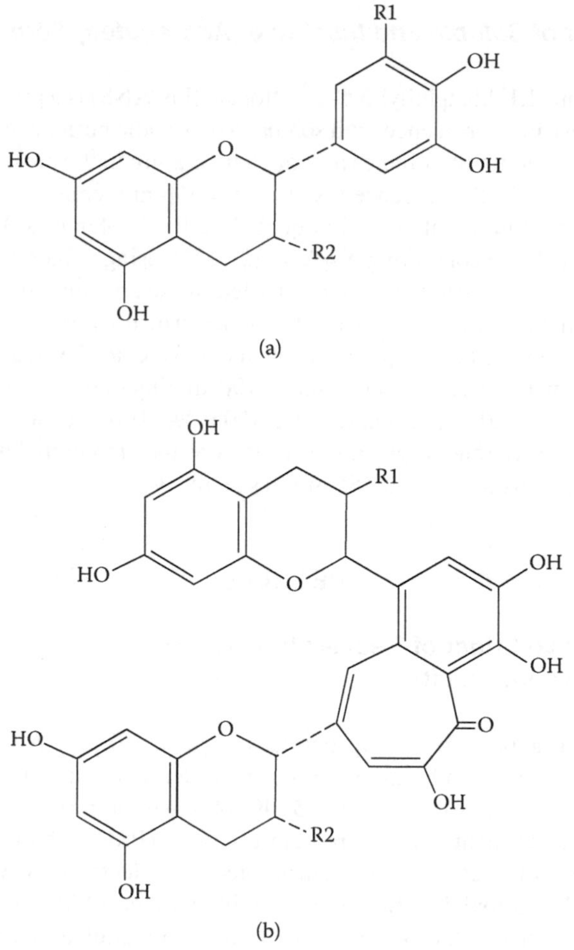

(a)

(b)

Figure 6.1 Comparative structures of main phenolic compounds derived from green (a) and black (b) tea.

effect of green and black tea extracts was shared by epigallocatechin gallate (EGCG, Figure 6.1), which appears to be the most potent green tea ingredient at 10 μM, and tends to be toxic at higher concentrations (20 μM) (data not shown). Epicatechin gallate (ECG), which represents approximately 5% of the total extract,[25] exerted somewhat fewer neuroprotective effects at 20 μM. In contrast, nongallate forms of catechins such as epicatechin (EC) and epigallocatechin (EGC) failed to display any protective effects against $A\beta_{25-35}$-induced toxicity.

The Sytox green assay revealed that the physiological fragment $A\beta_{1-42}$ (15 μM) displayed neurotoxic effects (27–45% increase in Sytox green fluorescence vs. control). The green (25 μg/ml) and black (5 μg/ml) tea extracts were able to completely block cell death produced by $A\beta_{1-42}$ (15 μM), as did the ginkgo biloba extract referred to as EGb 761 (100 μg/ml), a well-known standardized natural extract with purported beneficial clinical effects in AD patients.[26] Similar, albeit less neuroprotective, action was observed with the most abundant tea catechin EGCG (10 μM).

Finally, we tested the actions of other phenolic compounds derived from various sources including fruits, vegetables, and plants. Among those tested, piceatannol, a natural resveratrol analog, was the most potent, followed by morin and myricetin. In contrast, quercetin and kaempferol were ineffective. Moreover, phenolic acids—namely, tannic and gallic acids—were the only ones that were neuroprotective in our model, as summarized in Table 6.1.

Table 6.1   Summary of Effects of Tea Extracts and Phenolic Compounds against Toxicity Induced by Aβ Peptides in Rat Hippocampal Cell Cultures

Treatment	Neuroprotection
Green tea extract	+
Black tea extract	+
Epigallocatechin gallate	+
Epicatechin gallate	+
Epigallocatechin	−
Epicatechin	−
Resveratrol	+
Piceatannol	+
Quercetin	−
Kaempferol	−
Myricetin	+
Morin	+
Tannic acid	+
Gallic acid	+

Source: Taken from Bastianetto, S. et al., *Eur J Neurosci*, Jan, 23(1), 55–64, 2006; Ono, K. et al., *J Neurochem*, Oct, 87(1), 172–181, 2003; Ono, K. et al., *Biochim Biophys Acta*, Nov. 5, 1690(3), 193–202, 2004; and present chapter.

Neuroprotective Action of EGCG Does Not Involve Its Antioxidant Properties

Since free radical accumulation was proposed to mediate Aβ toxicity,[27] we studied the effects of EGCG on intracellular reactive oxygen species (ROS) using DCF assay. As expected, a 24-hour exposure to $A\beta_{1-42}$ resulted in a small but significant increase in DCF fluorescence (+18% relative to control), which was reduced by EGCG (10 μM) and by EC (10 μM), a tea catechin that failed to protect cells.

Inhibitory Action of Green Tea Catechins, Gallate Esters, and Other Polyphenols on Soluble and Insoluble Forms of Aβ

Since a co-treatment with EGCG displayed neuroprotective abilities against $A\beta_{1-42}$-induced toxicity, we hypothesized that it may directly interact with the amyloid peptide. Based on the purported fibril-destabilizing effects of various polyphenols,[20,28] we investigated the *in vitro* effect of various polyphenols on both soluble (nonaggregated) and insoluble (aged, aggregated) forms of Aβ using the Bis-ANS and ThT fluorescence assays, respectively. A 30-minute incubation of $A\beta_{1-42}$ (15 μM) resulted in an increase in Bis-ANS fluorescence (+ 35- to 75-fold relative to control), reflecting the presence of high amounts of soluble forms of $A\beta_{1-42}$. Increased fluorescence was diminished in the presence of green tea extract, EGCG, and ECG. In contrast, phenolic compounds that failed to protect cells (with the exception of resveratrol and morin), were not able to modulate Bis-ANS fluorescence.

A 24-hour incubation with a fresh solution of $A\beta_{1-42}$ (15 μM) increased ThT fluorescence by 30- to 50-fold relative to control. Phenolic compounds that displayed neuroprotective ability were able to abolish increase in ThT fluorescence assay, whereas EC and EGC were ineffective; results are summarized in Table 6.2.

Identification of [³H]-Resveratrol Binding Sites

We evaluated [³H]-resveratrol binding sites in rat brain subcellular fractions. Significant [³H]-resveratrol binding was detected in plasma membrane (PII fraction) and, to a lesser extent, in nuclear and large cellular components. Binding to the plasma membrane fraction was significantly reduced by pretreatment with trypsin, suggesting that specific [³H]-resveratrol binding sites are of a proteinaceous nature and are particularly enriched in the plasma membrane. Scatchard transformation of isotherm saturation binding experiments suggested that [³H]-resveratrol specifically binds to a single class of sites, with an apparent affinity of 220 ± 80 nM in the PII fraction.

Next we evaluated a series of resveratrol analogs and catechins for their ability to compete for specific [³H]-resveratrol binding in PII fraction. Interestingly, polyphenols that display neuroprotective action are the most potent ones to compete for specific [³H]-resveratrol binding with K_i values ranging from 25 nM (for EGCG) to 102 nM (for resveratrol), whereas molecules including EC and EGC were inactive.

Table 6.2 Comparative Effects of Tea Extracts
and Phenolic Compounds on Soluble
and Insoluble Forms of Aβ Peptides

Treatment	Soluble Forms of Aβ	Aβ Fibrils
Green tea extract	+	+
Black tea extract	ND	ND
Epigallocatechin gallate	+	+
Epicatechin gallate	+	−/+
Epigallocatechin	−	−
Epicatechin	−	−
Gallic acid	−	+
Resveratrol	−	+
Piceatannol	+	+
Quercetin	−	+
Myricetin	+	+
Morin	−	+

Note: ND: not determined.

Source: Taken from Bastianetto, S. et al., *Eur J Neurosci*, Jan,
23(1), 55–64, 2006; Ono, K. et al., *J Neurochem*, Oct,
87(1), 172–181, 2003; Ono, K. et al., *Biochem Biophys Acta*, Nov. 5, 1690(3), 193–202, 2004; and present chapter.

The affinity of polyphenols and various resveratrol analogs to compete for specific
[3H]-resveratrol binding correlated very well ($r = 0.74$) with their neuroprotective
activity against $A\beta_{25-35}$-induced toxicity in primary hippocampal cell cultures. This
suggests that the neuroprotective effect exerted by these phenolic compounds could
be mediated by a common mechanism involving specific polyphenol plasma membrane binding sites.

DISCUSSION

We have demonstrated that polyphenols such as resveratrol and tea catechins
gallate esters (i.e., ECG and EGCG) are able to protect cultured hippocampal cells
against Aβ-induced toxicity. These data are consistent with those previously reported
showing that polyphenol-derived extracts (particularly green tea) and their main
constituents display neuroprotective actions in various *in vitro* and animal models
of toxicity.[29,30] Moreover, these data suggest that intake of polyphenols consumed in
various forms (green and black teas, red wine, fruits, and vegetables) may attenuate
the toxic effects of accumulation of Aβ peptides involved in the neurodegenerative
process occurring in AD.[1]

Resveratrol, an active silbene from grapes, was shown to concentration-depend-
ently protect against Aβ-induced toxicity in cultured hippocampal neurons. The
mechanisms involved in the neuroprotective effects of resveratrol likely include PKC
as revealed by the inhibitory action of the potent PKC antagonist GF 109203X and

the stimulation of PKC phosphorylation by resveratrol. Moreover, resveratrol failed to modulate the phosphorylation of other kinases such as ERK1 and ERK2, in contrast to earlier results.[31] Taken together, our results suggest that the PKC pathway, but not MAP and Akt kinases, plays a major role in the neuroprotective properties of resveratrol against Aβ-induced toxicity in hippocampal neurons. Other mechanisms may also be involved since resveratrol has been shown to promote proteasome-dependent intracellular Aβ degradation[22] and to inhibit Aβ fibril formation,[32] in accordance with our present results.

Black and green tea extracts behave as potent plant extracts against Aβ toxicity, due to the presence of flavan-3-ols found predominantly as monomers and dimers in green and black tea, respectively.[25,33] Among flavan-3-ols monomers tested here, only EGCG and, to a lesser extent, ECG displayed strong neuroprotective activities, in accordance with previous studies.[12,14] Similar protective effects were also observed with theaflavins, which are flavan-3-ols dimers that are almost exclusively present in black tea.[25] The fact that these protective effects were observed only with EGCG and ECG, but not with EC and EGC, indicates that the esterification of the pyran hydroxyl group of catechins by gallic acid plays a key role in their neuroprotective activities. In support of this hypothesis, gallic acid significantly protected against Aβ peptide-induced toxicity.[11] Findings from DCF fluorescence assay indicate that EGCG was able to inhibit ROS accumulation generated by $Aβ_{1-42}$, as did EC, a green tea catechin that failed to be neuroprotective. Taken together, these data suggest that the antioxidant activities of EGCG are not significantly involved in its protective action against Aβ peptides in our model.

We then examined the role of various polyphenols in the formation of Aβ fibrils and soluble forms of $Aβ_{1-42}$. Globally, phenolic compounds that share their capacities to protect hippocampal cells inhibited Aβ fibril and/or oligomer formation. These data are in accordance with previous studies revealing that phenolic acids and polyphenols display anti-amyloidogenic and fibril-destabilizing activities.[13,20,21,28,32] Moreover, we have found that various polyphenols, including EGCG, have an inhibitory effect on nonfibrillar monomers and oligomers, including Aβ-derived diffusible ligands (ADDLs) that were suggested to mediate the neurotoxic effects of $Aβ_{1-42}$.[3] Taken together, these data suggest that the inhibitory action of polyphenols on Aβ fibril/oligomer formation contributes, at least in part, to their neuroprotective action against Aβ-induced neurotoxicity.

Finally, binding studies revealed the existence, at the level of the cell plasma membrane, of specific polyphenol binding sites in the rat brain. Structure–activity data support the hypothesis that these specific binding sites may mediate numerous biological effects of these polyphenols, including their neuroprotective abilities.

In summary, these findings demonstrate that the neuroprotective action of polyphenols—particularly tea catechin gallate esters—is partly due to their inhibitory action on Aβ oligomer and/or fibril formation. This supports the hypothesis of the purported preventive effects of moderate consumption of red wine and regular intake of tea, fruits, and vegetables against Alzheimer's disease and suggests that polyphenols may be useful neuroprotective agents.

ACKNOWLEDGMENT

This work was supported by research grants from the Canadian Institutes of Health Research (CIHR) to Rémi Quirion.

ABBREVIATIONS

Aβ: β-amyloid
AD: Alzheimer's disease
bis-ANS: 4,4′-dianilino-1,1′-binaphthyl-5,5′-disulfonate
DCF: dichlorofluorescein
EC: epicatechin
ECG: epicatechin gallate
EGC: epigallocatechin
EGCG: epigallocatechin gallate
EGb 761: gingko biloba extract
PKC: protein kinase C
ROS: reactive oxygen species
Th-T: thioflavin T

REFERENCES

1. Hardy, J., and Selkoe, D.J., The amyloid hypothesis of Alzheimer's disease: Progress and problems on the road to therapeutics. *Science*, Nov 1, 298(5595), 962–1044, 2002.
2. Terry, R.D., An honorable compromise regarding amyloid in Alzheimer disease. *Ann Neurol*, May, 49(5), 684, 2001.
3. Klein, W.L., ADDLs and protofibrils—The missing links? *Neurobiol Aging*, Mar–Apr, 23(2), 231–235, 2002.
4. Luchsinger, J.A., Tang, M.X., Siddiqui, M., Shea, S., and Mayeux, R., Alcohol intake and risk of dementia. *J Am Geriatr Soc*, Apr, 52(4), 540–546, 2004.
5. Orgogozo, J.M., Dartigues, J.F., Lafont, S., Letenneur, L., Commenges, D., Salomon, R., Renaud, S., and Breteler, M.B., Wine consumption and dementia in the elderly: A prospective community study in the Bordeaux area. *Rev Neurol*, Apr, 153(3), 185–192, 1997.
6. Pan, T., Jankovic, J., and Le, W., Potential therapeutic properties of green tea polyphenols in Parkinson's disease. *Drugs Aging*, 20(10), 711–721, 2003.
7. Dauchet, L., Amouyel, P., and Dallongeville, J., Fruit and vegetable consumption and risk of stroke: A meta-analysis of cohort studies. *Neurology*, Oct 25, 65(8), 1193–1197, 2005.
8. Dai, Q., Borenstein, A.R., Wu, Y., Jackson, J.C., and Larson, E.B., Fruit and vegetable juices and Alzheimer's disease: The Kame Project. *Am J Med*, Sep, 119(9), 751–759, 2006.
9. Commenges, D., Scotet, V., Renaud, S., Jacqmin-Gadda, H., Barberger-Gateau, P., and Dartigues, J.F., Intake of flavonoids and risk of dementia. *Eur J Epidemiol*, Apr, 16(4), 357–363, 2000.
10. Han, Y.S., Zheng, W.H., Bastianetto, S., Chabot, J.G., and Quirion, R., Neuroprotective effects of resveratrol against beta-amyloid-induced neurotoxicity in rat hippocampal neurons: Involvement of protein kinase C. *Br J Pharmacol*, Mar, 141(6), 997–1005, 2004.

11. Bastianetto, S., Yao, Z.X., Papadopoulos, V., and Quirion, R., Neuroprotective effects of green and black teas and their catechin gallate esters against beta-amyloid-induced toxicity. *Eur J Neurosci,* Jan, 23(1), 55–64, 2006.

12. Choi, Y.T., Jung, C.H., Lee, S.R., Bae, J.H., Baek, W.K., Suh, M.H., Park, J., Park, C.W., and Suh, S.I., The green tea polyphenol (–)-epigallocatechin gallate attenuates beta-amyloid-induced neurotoxicity in cultured hippocampal neurons. *Life Sci,* Dec 21, 70(5), 603–614, 2001.

13. Rezai-Zadeh, K., Shytle, D., Sun, N., Mori, T., Hou, H., Jeanniton, D., Ehrhart, J., Townsend, K., Zeng, J., Morgan, D., Hardy, J., Town, T., and Tan, J., Green tea epigallocatechin-3-gallate (EGCG) modulates amyloid precursor protein cleavage and reduces cerebral amyloidosis in Alzheimer transgenic mice. *J Neurosci,* Sep 21, 25(38), 8807–8814, 2005.

14. Levites, Y., Amit, T., Mandel, S., and Youdim, M.B., Neuroprotection and neurorescue against Abeta toxicity and PKC-dependent release of nonamyloidogenic soluble precursor protein by green tea polyphenol (–)-epigallocatechin-3-gallate. *FASEB J,* May, 17(8), 952–954, 2003.

15. Levites, Y., Amit, T., Youdim, M.B., and Mandel, S., Involvement of protein kinase C activation and cell survival/cell cycle genes in green tea polyphenol (–)-epigallocatechin 3-gallate neuroprotective action. *J Biol Chem,* Aug 23, 277(34), 30574–30580, 2002.

16. Le Bars, P.L., Kieser, M., and Itil, K.Z., A 26-week analysis of a double-blind, placebo-controlled trial of the ginkgo biloba extract EGb 761 in dementia. *Dement Geriatr Cogn Disord,* Jul–Aug, 11(4), 230–237, 2000.

17. Bastianetto, S., Ramassamy, C., Dore, S., Christen, Y., Poirier, J., and Quirion, R., The ginkgo biloba extract (EGb 761) protects hippocampal neurons against cell death induced by β-amyloid. *Eur J Neurosci,* Jun, 12(6), 1882–1890, 2000.

18. Yao, Z., Drieu, K., and Papadopoulos, V., The ginkgo biloba extract EGb 761 rescues the PC12 neuronal cells from beta-amyloid-induced cell death by inhibiting the formation of beta-amyloid-derived diffusible neurotoxic ligands. *Brain Res,* Jan 19, 889(1–2), 181–190, 2001.

19. Stackman, R.W., Eckenstein, F., Frei, B., Kulhanek, D., Nowlin, J., and Quinn, J.F., Prevention of age-related spatial memory deficits in a transgenic mouse model of Alzheimer's disease by chronic ginkgo biloba treatment. *Exp Neurol,* Nov, 184(1), 510–520, 2003.

20. Ono, K., Yoshiike, Y., Takashima, A., Hasegawa, K., Naiki, H., and Yamada, M., Potent anti-amyloidogenic and fibril-destabilizing effects of polyphenols *in vitro*: Implications for the prevention and therapeutics of Alzheimer's disease. *J Neurochem,* Oct, 87(1), 172–181, 2003.

21. Porat, Y., Abramowitz, A., and Gazit, E., Inhibition of amyloid fibril formation by polyphenols: Structural similarity and aromatic interactions as a common inhibition mechanism. *Chem Biol Drug Des,* Jan, 67(1), 27–37, 2006.

22. Marambaud, P., Zhao, H., and Davies, P., Resveratrol promotes clearance of Alzheimer's disease amyloid-β peptides. *J Biol Chem,* Nov 11, 280(45), 37377–37382, 2005.

23. Bastianetto, S., Zheng, W.H., and Quirion, R. Neuroprotective abilities of resveratrol and other red wine constituents against nitric oxide-related toxicity in cultured hippocampal neurons. *Br J Pharmacol,* Oct, 131(4), 711–720, 2000.

24. LeVine, H., 3rd, 4(′)-Dianilino-1,1(′)-binaphthyl-5,5(′)-disulfonate: Report on non-beta-sheet conformers of Alzheimer's peptide beta$_{1-40}$. *Arch Biochem Biophys,* Aug 1, 404(1), 106–115, 2002.

25. Del Rio, D., Stewart, A.J., Mullen, W., Burns, J., Lean, M.E., Brighenti, F., and Crozier, A., HPLC-MSn analysis of phenolic compounds and purine alkaloids in green and black tea. *J Agric Food Chem,* May 19, 52(10), 2807–2815, 2004.
26. Le Bars, P.L., Magnitude of effect and special approach to ginkgo biloba extract EGb 761 in cognitive disorders. *Pharmacopsychiatry,* Jun, 36 Suppl 1, S44–49, 2003.
27. Behl, C., Davis, J.B., Lesley, R., and Schubert, D., Hydrogen peroxide mediates amyloid beta protein toxicity. *Cell,* Jun 17, 77(6), 817–827, 1994.
28. Ono, K., Hasegawa, K., Naiki, H., and Yamada, M., Anti-amyloidogenic activity of tannic acid and its activity to destabilize Alzheimer's beta-amyloid fibrils *in vitro. Biochim Biophys Acta,* Nov. 5, 1690(3), 193–202, 2004.
29. Hong, J.T., Ryu, S.R., Kim, H.J., Lee, J.K., Lee, S.H., Kim, D.B., Yun, Y.P., Ryu, J.H., Lee, B.M., and Kim, P.Y., Neuroprotective effect of green tea extract in experimental ischemia-reperfusion brain injury. *Brain Res Bull,* Dec, 53(6), 743–749, 2000.
30. Skrzydlewska, E., Ostrowska, J., Farbiszewski, R., and Michalak, K. Protective effect of green tea against lipid peroxidation in the rat liver, blood serum and the brain. *Phytomedicine,* Apr, 9(3), 232–238, 2002.
31. Miloso, M., Bertelli, A.A., Nicolini, G., and Tredici, G., Resveratrol-induced activation of the mitogen-activated protein kinases, ERK1 and ERK2, in human neuroblastoma SH-SY5Y cells. *Neurosci Lett,* Apr 2, 264(1–3), 141–144, 1999.
32. Riviere, C., Richard, T., Quentin, L., Krisa, S., Merillon, J.M., and Monti, J.P., Inhibitory activity of stilbenes on Alzheimer's beta-amyloid fibrils *in vitro. Bioorg Med Chem,* Jan 15, 15(2), 1160–1167, 2007. Epub 2006 Oct 1.
33. Wang, X., Song, K.S., Guo, Q.X., and Tian, W.X., The galloyl moiety of green tea catechins is the critical structural feature to inhibit fatty-acid synthase. *Biochem Pharmacol,* Nov 15, 66(10), 2039–2047, 2003.

CHAPTER 7

Green Tea
Skin Care and Skin Diseases

Stephen D. Hsu

CONTENTS

INTRODUCTION

The orderly progression of normal epidermal keratinocytes results in the highly organized functional layers of the epidermis and skin barrier. However, in the epidermis of psoriasis and many other skin disorders, aberrant differentiation and hyperproliferation of epidermal keratinocytes, as well as inflammation, lead to skin lesions and a disrupted barrier characterized by an altered stratum corneum. A newly discovered pathological characteristic of psoriasis is the abnormal expression and processing of caspase 14, a member of the caspase family that is associated with epithelial cell differentiation, planned cell death, and barrier formation. We previously found that green tea polyphenols (GTPs) or the most abundant GTP, (–) -epigallocatechin-3-gallate (EGCG), are able to induce terminal differentiation in exponentially growing epidermal keratinocytes [1]. We recently discovered that (1) caspase 14 is induced by EGCG in exponentially growing normal human epidermal keratinocytes [2] and (2) human psoriatic tissues lack the nuclear localization of caspase 14 [3]. In addition to the prodifferentiation property, GTPs are known to possess anticancer, antioxidant, and anti-inflammatory effects.

These effects of GTPs may ultimately be used to improve skin conditions, protect the skin from damage caused by ultraviolet (UV) radiation, reduce symptoms of skin disorders, and help to heal wounds. However, information regarding the mechanisms by which GTPs accelerate differentiation in skin disorders remains to be determined, as well as the role of GTP-induced caspase 14 in epidermal keratinocytes. In a pilot study, we found that topical application of 0.5% GTPs significantly reduced the symptoms of epidermal pathology in flaky skin mice, a model for human psoriasis, in which proliferating cell nuclear antigen (PCNA) expression was reduced and caspase 14 appeared to be processed and localized in the nucleus. Since current treatment of psoriasis is often associated with toxicity and side effects, our results suggest that GTPs may provide a nontoxic alternative therapy for treatment of skin disorders such as psoriasis. Based on these observations, we hypothesize that topical application of GTPs or EGCG will protect the epidermis from symptoms associated with psoriasis by attenuating three keratinocyte-based mechanisms of pathogenesis: aberrant caspase 14 expression/processing, inflammation, and hyperproliferation. This chapter describes our investigations to explore the mechanisms by which GTPs protect the epidermal keratinocytes in a mouse model for skin disorders, and the role of caspase 14 in GTP-induced acceleration of cell differentiation, cornification, and barrier formation.

THE ORIGIN OF GREEN TEA

The tea plant (*camellia sinensis*) has existed in nature for 60–70 million years. The earliest Chinese literature indicates that the Chinese cultivated tea plants thousands of years ago. In the Chinese legend, the Emperor Shen-Nung (2737–2697 B.C.) placed camellia blossom tips into a cup of boiled water and pronounced the beverage healing and refreshing. The first documented medicinal use of tea stated in *Shen-Nung's Book of Herbal Medicine* that "Shen-Nung tasted one hundred types of herbs each day and was intoxicated seventy-two times, each time he was able to revitalize by drinking tea." In the most famous Chinese herbal medicine textbook, written by Li Shi-Zhen (1518–1593), tea was described as able to bring down fever and brighten the eyes. Thus, tea initially was utilized as a type of herbal medicine for detoxification.

As a beverage, tea consumption began in earnest about 200 B.C., and then popularized when it was said to cure General Zhu Ge Liang (181–234 A.D.), who introduced tea consumption to ethnic minority Chinese in the southwest area of the country. Today, those people still call him the "Tea God." During the Tang Dynasty (618–907 A.D.), tea became an essential component of Chinese culture due to the first book describing in detail the use of tea; 28-year-old Chinese author Lu Yu (733–804 A.D.) published the book *Cha Jing* (literally, *The Book of Tea*), systematically chronicling the planting, processing, preparation, and consumption of the tea now referred to as green tea.

Japan was the first country to import the tea plant and tea culture from China, probably during the Tang Dynasty, when the countries exchanged Buddhist monks. Japan's "tea culture," which incorporated cultural, spiritual, and ceremonial activities into the consumption of the beverage, originated in China. The humble beverage began competing with romance as the inspiration for countless poems, songs, and fine arts that are still thriving in Asian countries.

After the Tang Dynasty, tea plant seeds from China were spread into more than 50 countries. Today, tea is the most popular beverage in the world, with black tea accounting for 78% of the consumption and green tea most of the remainder. Tea production worldwide exceeds 2.9 million tons a year, with 80% produced in Asia. In the United States, overall tea consumption has increased 300% in 10 years— the same time period that saw the country's first *decline* in per capita cancer rates. During the past 20 years, green tea consumption became more popular in the West due to the recognition of health benefits of catechins, also referred to as green tea polyphenols. Therefore, green tea is now "rediscovered" for medicinal use to prevent, delay, and treat human diseases.

Green Tea Polyphenols

Green tea polyphenols are found in the leaves of the tea plant (*Camellia sinensis*). Processing of green tea by heating briefly and drying the tea leaves inactivate polyphenol oxidase, therefore preserving the GTPs from oxidation and polymerization. The four major polyphenols present in green tea leaves are (–)-epicatechin (EC), (–)-epigallocatechin (EGC), (–)-epicatechin-3-gallate (ECG), and (–)-epigallocatechin-3-gallate (EGCG), which is the most abundant and has been well characterized as the most potent GTP [3–6].

Anticancer Properties

Cancer of the epidermis is the most common cancer type in the United States, according to the Centers for Disease Control and Prevention [7]. Excluding melanoma,

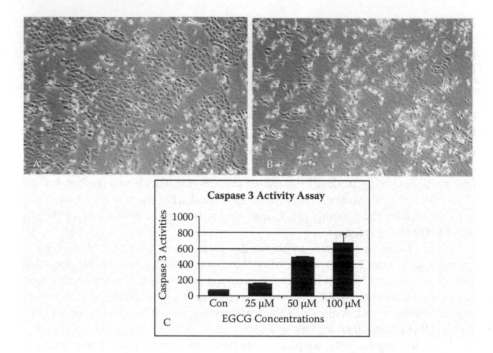

Figure 7.1 Activation of caspase 3–mediated apoptosis in skin cancer cells A-431 by EGCG. A. Control cells without EGCG exposure. B. Cells exposed to 50 μM for 24 h. C. EGCG dose-dependently induced the activation of caspase 3 in A-431 cells during a 24-h period. The caspase 3 activity measured by the cleavage of a substrate peptide increased by two-, six-, and ninefold compared to control when cells were exposed to 25, 50, and 100 μM of EGCG, respectively.

the incidence of basal cell carcinoma (BCC) and squamous cell carcinoma (SCC) of skin is estimated to exceed one million cases per year [8]. Squamous cell carcinoma is also a major type of cancer found in the neck and the oral cavity. Many epithelial-derived cancers lack the response to differentiation signals. This inability to respond to differentiation signals is due to alterations in gene expression caused by accumulation of gene defects. GTPs are known antioxidants that also possess anticancer activities. One of the unique characteristics of GTPs is that they selectively induce growth arrest and apoptosis in many types of tumor cells while protecting certain normal epithelial cells [6,9–14]. For example, EGCG at a topically achievable concentration of 50 μM was able to induce caspase 3-mediated apoptosis in skin cancer cells A431 within 24 hours (Figure 7.1).

Prodifferentiation Properties

GTPs and EGCG in particular are able to activate a pathway for cell differentiation in normal human epidermal keritinocytes (NHEKs). In contrast to tumor cells, NHEKs undergo accelerated differentiation when exposed to EGCG, which is associated with induction of p57/KIP2, a cyclin-dependent kinase inhibitor involved in cell growth and differentiation [1,15].

We found that GTPs or EGCG, at a topically achievable range, selectively induced caspase 3–dependent apoptosis in tumor cells, whereas NHEKs showed elevated p57/ KIP2 expression and underwent terminal differentiation in response to EGCG, without activation of caspase 3 [1,15–17]. Results from our previous gene microarray analysis also support the proposed model of a green tea–activated novel differentiation pathway and the inhibitory effect of EGCG on autoantigens [18,19]. We further investigated the relationship between EGCG and the expression caspase 14, a protein involved in terminal differentiation of epidermal keratinocytes, in an *in vitro* tumor versus normal system: NHEKs, OSC2 (an oral squamous cell carcinoma line), and clones derived from OSC2 cells that overexpress p57/KIP2. The results demonstrate that EGCG coordinately activates the expression of p57 and caspase 14 in NHEKs, which facilitates terminal differentiation in these cells [2]. In addition, we found that human psoriatic tissue lacks significant nuclear localization of caspase 14 [2,3]. Psoriasis has been considered to be a disease with both immunological and epidermal abnormalities that is characterized by inflammation, hyperproliferation, and hypodifferentiation, leading to aberrant barrier formation. In this regard, our observation that psoriatic keratinocytes exhibit aberrant expression and/or nuclear localization of caspase 14 may explain the failure of cornification and appropriate barrier formation in psoriatic epidermis.

Anti-inflammatory Properties

In addition to the anticancer, prodifferentiation, and antioxidant effects, GTPs/ EGCG also possess the ability to [18 21]

inhibit cyclooxygenase (COX) 2, tumor necrosis factor (TNF)-α, interferon (IFN)-γ, inducible nitric oxide synthase (iNOS), and phase I and phase II enzymes
inhibit inflammation-related responses such as interleukin (IL)-1, IL-10, and IL-12 release
inhibit IL-1β-induced metalloproteinase (MMP)-1 and MMP-13
suppress the caspase 3–mediated apoptosis pathway
inhibit autoantigen expression

These properties could provide additional preventive/therapeutic effects toward psoriatic lesions. Thus, the potential use of green tea constituents as an alternative nontoxic preventive agent or therapeutic component to treat psoriasis and other skin disorders needs to be explored.

The Epidermis

In human skin, keratinocytes within the epidermis exist in various stages of differentiation corresponding to different epidermal layers [22,23]. Cells of the basal layer (stratum germinatum) at the dermal–epidermal junction continuously proliferate to regenerate and restore cells that are shed to the environment from the cornified layer (stratum corneum). As the daughter cells migrate up through the epidermal layers, they first gradually undergo growth arrest, followed by expression of keratins 1 and 10 in the stratum spinosum (spinous layer). In the next layer, the stratum granulosum (granular layer) and late markers of keratinocyte differentiation, including filaggrin and other structural proteins, are expressed and lipogenesis occurs. Late in this stage of keratinocyte differentiation, the cells are denucleated. In addition, transglutaminase, the enzyme that cross-links the structural proteins into the cornified envelope, is activated. Finally, the keratinocytes undergo epidermal-specific planned cell death to form the stratum corneum, which serves as a semipermeable barrier to mechanical injury, microbial invasion, and water loss. The entire epidermis turns over in 1–2 months, although the transit time of keratinocytes may be lengthened or shortened in various disease states.

The Stratum Corneum

The stratum corneum consists of denucleated corneocytes filled with cross-linked proteins, while the intercellular space is occupied by lipids synthesized prior to and during cornification [24]. Formation of this barrier relies on the cornification of epidermal keratinocytes, which undergo growth arrest, terminal differentiation, and an epidermal-specific cell death, referred to as "planned cell death" [25]. Abnormalities in any of these programmed events may lead to epidermal disorders such as psoriasis, atopic dermatitis, and cancer. However, biological events that enable basal cells (stem cells) to proliferate, differentiate, and commit planned cell death are still poorly understood [10]. The keratinocyte differentiation process can be stimulated by prodifferentiation agents such as extracellular calcium and 1, 25-dihydroxy cholecalciferol (referred to as "vitamin D3" hereafter) [23]. Aberrant or absent differentiation can be found in other skin disorders such as atopic keratosis, seborrheic keratosis, and rosacea.

Psoriasis

Psoriasis is a skin disorder that affects up to 2% of the U.S. population. The pathogenesis of psoriasis, which has epidermal and immunity components, is still under investigation. About 4.5 million Americans suffer from this disease, often with a significant negative impact on their quality of life (National Psoriasis Foundation 2001 Benchmark Survey on Psoriasis and Psoriatic Arthritis). Psoriasis is involved in aberrant differentiation and hyperproliferation of epidermal keratinocytes, as well as inflammation, leading to skin lesions and a disrupted barrier characterized by an altered stratum corneum. In psoriatic epidermis, the keratinocytes do not undergo the denucleation process, but continue to proliferate. The most common treatments currently used include phototherapies, potent topical steroids, oral retinoids, immunosuppressive agents such as methotrexate or cyclosporine, and newer biological agents that block cytokine or cellular immune factors [43]. All are associated with untoward side effects, and the biological agents must be given parenterally and are very expensive. A combination of psoralen and ultraviolet A (UVA), referred to as PUVA therapy, has been used for treatment of psoriasis to reduce the toxicity caused by systemic drugs [25]. However, prolonged treatment with PUVA increases the risk of skin cancer, especially squamous cell carcinoma [26]. Vitamin D3 and its analogs have been recently used as another option, but they can cause hypermineralization if overdosed. Clearly, more work is required to identify treatments that are safe, effective, convenient to administer, and reasonably priced.

Caspase 14

Identified in 1998 from murine tissues, caspase 14 is expressed only in epithelial tissues, especially in the differentiating epidermis [27–29]. The human caspase 14 gene is located on chromosome 19p13.1 and consists of seven exons. RNA splicing results in two mRNA species, referred to as caspase 14a and caspase 14b, which translate into two caspase 14 protein variants [30]. The unprocessed caspase 14 protein, with a molecular weight of 28 kDa, is not catalytically active. The 17- and 11-kDa subunits found in the stratum corneum of normal human epidermis result from proteolysis and are able to specifically cleave tetrapeptide substrates; but 28-kD caspase 14 is predominant in human psoriatic plaques, where cornification and nuclear destruction are absent [31]. Thus, the activity of caspase 14 is associated with cornification and nuclear destruction of the epidermis. However, the proteolytic enzyme responsible for caspase 14 processing is unknown, as are the endogenous substrates. Unlike the other caspases, caspase 14 is not involved in the pro-apoptotic caspase cascade, but is associated with terminal differentiation of NHEKs and barrier formation [32–34].

In addition to the epidermis, caspase 14 expression also was found in the choroid plexus, hair follicles, retinal pigment epithelium, and thymic Hassall's bodies—all tissues involved in barrier functioning [35]. Interestingly, caspase 14 protein is absent from oral epithelium, which lacks stratum corneum [33]. In the epidermis, induction of caspase 14 at the transcriptional level was noted during stratum corneum formation [30]. Caspase 14 in its various forms is in the cytoplasm and nucleus of the granular layer, in the nuclear remnants of the transitional layer of the epidermis, and in the stratum corneum [36], where caspase 14 is processed to 17- and 11-kD subunits [31]. The co-localization of caspase 14 and the nuclear remnants suggests a possible link between caspase 14 and nuclear breakdown in keratinocytes during terminal differentiation. Caspase 14 expression was diminished with inhibition of cell differentiation by retinoic acid [37]. Therefore, caspase 14 is believed to facilitate epidermal differentiation, possibly activating planned cell death and cornification of the epidermis to form the skin barrier [31]. In contrast, in pathological conditions such as psoriasis, in which cornification is interrupted, the normal expression and processing patterns of caspase 14 are absent [31,33].

EXPERIMENTAL RESULTS

EGCG Specifically Induced Caspase 14 Expression in NHEKs within 24 Hours

NHEKs were exposed to EGCG in eight-well chamberslides, followed by immunocytochemistry using rabbit anti-caspase 14 antibody (Santa Cruz, H-99). The results showed that caspase 14 protein was almost undetectable in control samples without

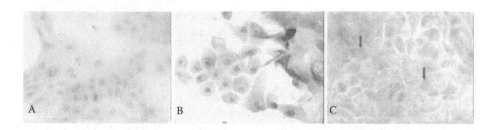

Figure 7.2 A. Immunostaining of caspase 14 in exponentially growing NHEKs (400×).
B. NHEKs treated with 50 μM EGCG for 24 h (400×). C. Confluent OSC2 cells (400×). Pre-
immune rabbit serum was used as negative control (data not shown), and cell nuclei were
counterstained with Mayer's hematoxylin.

EGCG exposure, which exhibited blue nuclei (Figure 7.2A). NHEKs incubated with
50 μ*M* EGCG for 24 hours showed a large amount of caspase 14 staining in both the
cytosol and nuclei, suggesting caspase 14 protein accumulated with EGCG treatment
and entered the nuclei (Figure 7.2B). OSC2 cells (a human oral carcinoma cell line)
exhibited basal cytosolic caspase 14 (arrows) staining, as shown in Figure 7.2C. We
further examined caspase 14 expression in A431 (a human epidermoid cancer cell
line), OSC2, and HSG (a human salivary gland cancer cell line) cells, with or without
EGCG exposure, by Western blotting with the same antibody and found that caspase
14 protein was not expressed in A431 or HSG cell lines, whereas OSC2 cells exhibited a low basal level of caspase 14 (data not shown, [44]).

EGCG Induced mRNA and Protein Levels of Caspase 14 in NHEKs

To determine the time course of EGCG-activated caspase 14 mRNA accumulation, total RNA samples were collected at 0, 0.5, 2, 6, 8, 12, 20, and 24 hours after
exposure to 50 μ*M* EGCG. The RNA species were analyzed by semiquantitative
RT-PCR using GAPDH as an internal control. The caspase 14 mRNA peaked at
12 hours [2]. To determine the protein levels of caspase 14 in response to EGCG,
cell lysates were prepared from NHEKs exposed to 50 μ*M* EGCG for 0, 4, 6, 8, 12,
20, and 24 hours prior to Western blot analysis using a rabbit polyclonal anti-caspase
14 and antihuman actin antibodies. The anti-caspase 14 antibody was raised against
amino acids 24–122, mapping near the N terminus of human caspase 14 protein
(Santa Cruz, H-99). In addition, it specifically recognized human caspase 14 protein
expressed in tumor cells by a caspase 14 cDNA construct (pCMV, obtained from
Origene). Protein levels of caspase 14 gradually increased from 4 to 12 hours, and
peaked at 20 hours, equivalent to a fivefold increase related to control normalized
with actin [2].

Psoriatic Tissue Lacks Normal Expression Pattern and Nuclear Localization of Caspase 14

Normal human epidermis exhibited homogeneous caspase 14 staining in spinous
and granular layers and moderate staining in the basal layer, with evidence of nuclear

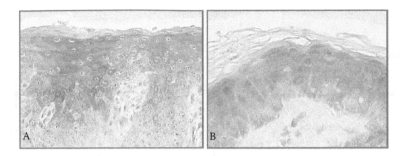

Figure 7.3 A. Human psoriatic tissue (200×). B. Normal human skin (200×). Both samples were immunostained with caspase 14 antibody. Punch biopsies (4 mm) of normal and psoriatic skin samples were obtained from different patients who provided written, informed consent under an IRB-approved protocol. Samples were fixed in 10% neutral-buffered formalin, paraffin embedded, cut to 5-µm sections, and stained with caspase 14 antibody by immunohistochemistry.

staining (Figure 7.3B). In contrast, the psoriasis samples exhibited moderate caspase 14 staining without significant nuclear localization of caspase 14 (Figure 7.3A).

Inhibition of MAPK Pathways Leads to Inhibition of EGCG-Induced Caspase 14 Expression

Our recent data demonstrated that while EGCG-induced p57 expression is strictly associated with the activation of the p38 mitogen-activated protein kinase (MAPK) pathway, caspase 14 expression activated by EGCG relies on either p38 or Jun N terminal kinase (JNK) activity. Inhibition of p38 suppressed both p57 and caspase 14 expression in NHEKs, while inhibition of JNK suppressed caspase 14 expression, but not p57. A MAPK/extracellular signal-regulated kinase kinase (MEK) inhibitor had no effect on the expression of either protein. This result suggests that EGCG induces caspase 14 via the p38 and JNK MAPK pathways (data not shown, [44]).

Transfection of Caspase 14 cDNA Altered Tumor Cell Behavior

A caspase 14–expressing vector pCMV/C14 from Origene (Rockville, Maryland) was transfected into OSC2 cells, as indicated in Figure 7.4A. Expression of caspase 14 resulted in the inhibitory effect of caspase 14 on OSC2 cell growth (Figure 7.4B). The EGCG-induced, caspase 3–mediated apoptosis was still observed in these caspase 14–expressing cells (Figure 7.4C). These results indicated that expression of exogenous caspase 14 inhibited OSC2 cell growth by approximately 25%, and EGCG effectively induced caspase 3–mediated apoptosis in caspase 14–expressing OSC2 cells. These data support our hypothesis that restoration of caspase 14 expression in tumor cells could alter cell behavior. This vector was also transfected into A431 cells, and restoration of caspase 14 in A431 cells resulted in growth inhibition and reduced tumorigenicity *in vivo* (data not shown, [45]).

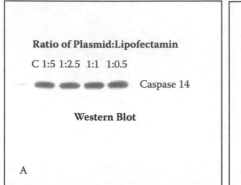

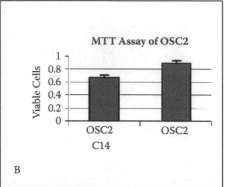

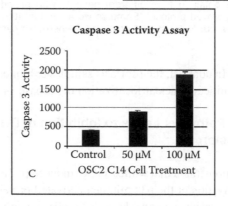

Figure 7.4   A. pCMV plasmid containing caspase 14 cDNA was transfected into OSC2 cells. The control cells (C, first lane) express small amounts of endogenous caspase 14. B. The growth of caspase 14–expressing OSC2 cells (OSC2 C14) was significantly slower than that of the parental cells. C. OSC2 caspase 14–expressing cells exhibit a basal level of caspase 3 activity, which was activated by EGCG in a dose-dependent manner.

GTPs Prevented Psoriasiform Lesions in a Pilot Study Using Flaky Skin Mice, a Model of Human Psoriasis

To investigate whether topical application of GTPs can prevent the development of psoriasiform lesions in flaky skin mice, animals were purchased from Jackson Laboratories (CByJ.A-fsn/+/J, 001723) at the age of 3 weeks. Six mice were randomly assigned to two groups. One group was bathed with warm water (37°C) 5 days/week. The other group was bathed with warm water containing 0.5% GTPs (37°C). At the age of 11 weeks, the animals in the water-treated group had developed skin lesions, but the animals in the water–GTP-treated group did not develop such skin lesions (Figure 7.5). At the end of week 13, animals were euthanized and skin samples were collected. The skin samples were fixed and either stained using a standard hematoxylin and eosin (H&E) method, or immunostained with antibodies against caspase 14 and against the PCNA. Figure 7.6 shows H&E-stained skin sections at 5 μm thick.

Water Only   **Water + GTPs**

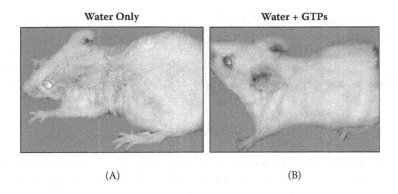

(A)   (B)

Figure 7.5 Flaky skin mice treated with a daily water bath (A) or a water–GTP bath (B) until the animals reached the age of 12 weeks, when the photo was taken. Skin samples were collected 1 week after this photo was taken.

(A)   (B)

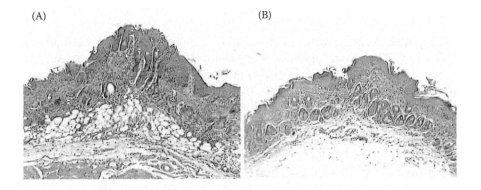

Figure 7.6 Flaky skin mouse skin samples stained by a standard H&E method. (A). The water-treated skin section shows marked hyperkeratosis, mild parakeratosis, modest acanthosis, elongated rete ridges, and modest dermal inflammation, consistent with psoriatic-like dermatitis. B. The water–GTE-treated skin section shows slight hyperkeratosis, no parakeratosis, mild acanthosis, no elongated rete ridges, and mild dermal inflammation (100× magnification).

The water-treated sample exhibits inflammation and increased thickness, while the water–GTP-treated sample has significantly less inflammation and thickness.

Immunostaining was performed on the skin samples from water-treated and water–GTE-treated flaky skin mice using caspase 14 antibody or proliferating cell nuclear antigen (PCNA) antibody. Nuclear caspase 14 staining appeared in the junction of the granular layer and the cornified layer in the water–GTE-treated sample. Immunostaining for PCNA, a marker for cell proliferation, was localized primarily in the basal layer of the water–GTE-treated sample, but the water-treated sample exhibited staining in suprabasal layers (data not shown, [44]).

Western blot results of these skin samples suggest that caspase 14 is predominantly present in water-treated skin as the catalytically inactive 30-kD form of mouse caspase 14, but the water–GTP-treated skin showed significantly higher levels of the catalytically active the 17-kD subunit. Since the 17-kD subunit is associated with the cornified layer and human psoriatic plaques have predominantly the 28-kD caspase 14 [31], this result suggests that cornification is more active in the water–GTP-treated skin. Results of the PCNA western blot confirmed the immunostaining result, where PCNA level was reduced in water–GTP-treated skin samples (data not shown, [44]).

DISCUSSION

Many skin disorders are associated with at least one of the characteristics of inflammation, oxidative stress, hyperproliferation, hypodifferentiation, infection, apoptosis, and autoimmune reactions. GTPs are uniquely positioned to antagonize these conditions with anti-inflammatory, antioxidant, antimicrobial, prodifferentiation, anti-apoptosis, and inhibition of autoantigen properties. Thus, many skin conditions, including autoimmune-induced lupus and psoriasis, wounds created by trauma or infections, damage induced by environmental factors such as UVB, and seborrheic dermatitis (dandruff), could be treated or managed by topical application of GTPs.

Regulation of cell growth and acceleration of differentiation in epidermal keratinocytes by GTPs would improve skin conditions, enhance wound healing, and restore skin barrier. Only certain epithelial tissues associated with barriers express significant levels of caspase 14 [33,36]. Tumors derived from the epithelial tissues of the cervix, ovary, breast, stomach, and colon exhibit altered expression of caspase 14 [38]. Our studies demonstrated that epithelial cancers derived from oral epithelium (OSC2), the salivary gland (HSG), and the epidermis (A431) do not express significant levels of caspase 14, nor do exponentially growing NHEKs (Figure 7.2). Exogenous caspase 14 expression leads to growth inhibition and reduced tumorigenicity in OSC2 and A431 cells (Figure 7.4, [45]). This evidence suggests that restoration of caspase 14 expression may alter cancer cell behavior by reducing the tumorigenicity of cancer cells, possibly through a differentiation mechanism. When NHEKs undergo EGCG-induced differentiation, caspase 14 levels are significantly elevated [2,18] (Figure 7.2B). These observations suggest that induction of caspase 14 expression by EGCG is associated with accelerated epithelial cell terminal differentiation.

In psoriatic epidermis, expression and processing of caspase 14 are altered. In comparison to normal epidermis, psoriatic epidermis is characterized by inflammation, hyperproliferation, hypodifferentiation, and aberrant cornification [25]. We found that EGCG-induced differentiation is associated with coordinated p57 and caspase 14 expression in NHEKs [2]. Our results obtained from recent studies suggests that EGCG-induced NHEK differentiation relies on, at least in part, the MAPK pathways. The p38 MAPK pathway is essential for EGCG-induced expression of involucrin, a marker for NHEK differentiation [39]. Similarly, EGCG-induced caspase 14 protein expression is mediated via both the p38 and JNK MAPK pathways, whereas p57 expression is associated only with the p38 MAPK pathway (data not shown [46]). These results suggest that inhibition of the p38 or JNK MAPK pathways could alter the cornification process and lead to interruption of the skin barrier, as shown in Jun knockout mice [40]. Thus, the p38 and JNK pathways used by GTPs for signal transduction, as well as the downstream transcription factors of these pathways, are essential for homeostasis of the epidermis.

Since caspase 14 plays an important role in epidermal keratinocyte terminal differentiation and denucleation, the effect of topical application of GTPs, with 40% EGCG, on the psoriasis symptoms in flaky skin mice was tested in this *in vivo* pilot study. The rationale for using GTPs instead of purified EGCG is that GTPs are naturally available without any chemical or compositional modification.

The epidermis of the flaky skin mice (Jackson lab, CByJ.A-fsn/J) exhibits hyperproliferation, aberrant differentiation, and inflammation after the onset of symptoms (when they are 4–5 weeks old). The autosomal recessive gene mutation in these animals is referred to as the flaky skin mouse mutation, *fsn*. The *fsn/fsn* mice are normal at birth except for hypochronic anemia. Before adulthood (8 weeks of age), they develop hyperkeratotic plaques and acanthosis, associated with thickened epidermis, a scarcity of hair, scale accumulation, and abnormal nail growth [41]. A large number of macrophages and mast cells can be observed at the dermal–epidermal junction, while neutrophils are found in the epidermis [41]. Skin grafts from the *fsn/fsn* mouse to athymic nude mice maintain the psoriasiform phenotype, associated with elevated DNA synthesis [42]. This evidence indicates that epidermal keratinocytes are essential for the pathogenesis of the psoriasiform phenotype manifested by the *fsn* mutation.

Histological analyses showed that the water-treated skin samples from these mice exhibited marked hyperkeratosis, mild parakeratosis, modest acanthosis, elongated rete ridges, and modest dermal inflammation—characteristics consistent with a psoriatic-like dermatitis (Figure 7.6A). In contrast, GTP-treated skin samples exhibited slight hyperkeratosis, no parakeratosis, mild acanthosis, no elongated rete ridges, and mild dermal inflammation (Figure 7.6B). Collectively, these results suggest that topical application of 0.5% GTPs can reduce the severity of psoriasis-like symptoms, both in terms of gross morphology and at the level of expression and localization of caspase 14 and PCNA.

Despite the encouraging results from our and others' studies, topical application of GTPs should not rely solely on fresh preparations carried out every day in the laboratories. It is important to develop topical preparations readily available for daily consumption. However, there are major problems that may prevent the use of GTP-containing products for everyday application. Since GTPs are highly water soluble and strong antioxidants, they are oxidized rapidly to form less active polymers in aqueous preparations containing oxygen. In addition, since GTPs are water soluble and the epidermis is waterproof, preparations containing GTPs may not deliver sufficient amounts of GTPs into the progressing keratinocytes in the epidermis. These issues must be addressed before chemically stable and penetrating formulations of GTPs can be successfully developed.

CONCLUSION

Our pilot study using the psoriasis mouse model demonstrates that, in psoriatic epidermis, GTPs restored, in part, the skin barrier by (1) reducing histological abnormalities, (2) promoting proteolytic processing of the 30-kD mouse caspase 14 into the 17-kD catalytically active enzyme, and (3) regulating cell growth by modulating PCNA expression. Our cell-based studies indicate that MAPK pathways upstream of Jun transcription factors are essential to skin homeostasis, and EGCG selectively activates p38 and JNK MAPK pathways to induce p57 and caspase 14, a protein needed for terminal differentiation and barrier formation. These data suggest that GTPs activate specific signal transduction pathways to regulate gene expression to accelerate terminal differentiation in the epidermis, in addition to their anticancer, antioxidant, and anti-inflammatory effects. These effects not only are beneficial to many skin disorders, but also may provide anti-aging results. Therefore, a popular beverage, green tea, is rediscovered to possess many preventive and therapeutic values for modern day medicinal application. Further investigation is needed to delineate fully the signal transduction pathways activated by GTPs/EGCG that regulate gene expression, leading to reduced inflammation, hyperproliferation, and hypo-differentiation. In conclusion, our results suggest that GTPs, a nontoxic plant-derived extract of green tea leaves, could be potentially useful in treating skin conditions such as psoriasis and help to protect the skin from various damage caused by either intrinsic or environmental factors.

REFERENCES

1. Hsu, S. et al. Tea polyphenols induce differentiation and proliferation in epidermal keratinocytes. *J Pharmacol Exp Ther.* 306, 29, 2003.
2. Hsu, S. et al. Green tea polyphenol-induced epithelial cell terminal differentiation is associated with coordinated expression of p57/KIP2 and caspase 14. *J Pharmacol Exp Ther.* 312, 884, 2005.
3. Walsh, D. et al. Psoriasis is characterized by altered epidermal expression of caspase 14, a novel regulator of keratinocyte terminal differentiation and barrier formation. *J Dermatol Sci.* 37, 61, 2005.
4. Katiyar, S.K. et al. Green tea polyphenols: DNA photodamage and photoimmunology. *J Photochem Photobiol B.* 65, 109, 2001.
5. Mukhtar, H. and Ahmad, N. Tea polyphenols: Prevention of cancer and optimizing health. *Am J Clin Nutr.* 71, 1698S, 2000.
6. Yang, C.S., Maliakal, P., and Meng, X. Inhibition of carcinogenesis by tea. *Annu Rev Pharmacol Toxicol.* 42, 25, 2002.
7. Preventing skin cancer: Findings of the Task Force on Community Preventive Services on Reducing Exposure to Ultraviolet Light. *CDC: Morbidity Mortality Weekly Rep.* 52(RR-15), 2003.
8. American Cancer Society. *Cancer facts & figures 2002.* Atlanta: American Cancer Society, 2002.

9. Adhami, V.M., Ahmad, N., and Mukhtar, H. Molecular targets for green tea in prostate cancer prevention. *J Nutr.* 133, 2417, 2003.
10. Balasubramanian, S., Efimova, T., and Eckert, R.L. Green tea polyphenol stimulates a Ras, MEKK1, MEK3, and p38 cascade to increase activator protein 1 factor-dependent involucrin gene expression in normal human keratinocytes. *J Biol Chem.* 277, 1828, 2002.
11. Hsu, S. et al. Chemoprevention of oral cancer by green tea. *Gen Dent.* 50, 140, 2002.
12. Hsu, S. et al. A mechanism-based *in vitro* anticancer drug screening approach for phenolic phytochemicals. *Assay Drug Dev Technol.* 1, 611, 2003.
13. Kazi, A. et al. Potential molecular targets of tea polyphenols in human tumor cells: Significance in cancer prevention. *In Vivo.* 16, 397, 2002.
14. Yamamoto, T. et al. Green tea polyphenol causes differential oxidative environments in normal vs. malignant cells. *J Pharmacol Exp Ther.* 307, 230, 2003.
15. Hsu, S. et al. Chemopreventive effects of green tea polyphenols correlate with reversible induction of p57 expression. *Anticancer Res.* 21, 3743, 2001.
16. Hsu, S. et al. Green tea polyphenol targets the mitochondria in tumor cells inducing caspase 3-dependent apoptosis. *Anticancer Res.* 23, 1533, 2003.
17. Hsu, S. et al. Induction of p57 is required for cell survival when exposed to green tea polyphenols. *Anticancer Res.* 22, 4115, 2002.
18. Hsu, S. Green tea and the skin. *J Am Acad Dermatol.* 52, 1049, 2005.
19. Hsu, S. et al. Inhibition of autoantigen expression by (–)-epigallocatechin-3-gallate (the major constituent of green tea) in normal human cells. *J Pharmacol Exp Ther.* 315, 805, 2005
20. Ahmed, S. et al. Green tea polyphenol epigallocatechin-3-gallate (EGCG) differentially inhibits interleukin-1 beta-induced expression of matrix metalloproteinase-1 and -13 in human chondrocytes. *J Pharmacol Exp Ther.* 308, 767, 2004.
21. Tedeschi, E. et al. Green tea inhibits human inducible nitric-oxide synthase expression by down-regulating signal transducer and activator of transcription-1alpha activation. *Mol Pharmacol.* 65, 111, 2004.
22. Bikle, D.D. et al. Calcium- and vitamin D-regulated keratinocyte differentiation. *Mol Cell Endocrinol.* 177, 161, 2001.
23. Bollag, W.B. and Bollag, R.J. 1,25-Dihydroxyvitamin D(3), phospholipase D and protein kinase C in keratinocyte differentiation. *Mol Cell Endocrinol.* 177, 173, 2001.
24. Madison, K.C. Barrier function of the skin: "La raison d'etre" of the epidermis. *J Invest Dermatol.* 121, 231, 2003.
25. Nickoloff, B.J. et al. Life and death signaling pathways contributing to skin cancer. *J Invest Dermatol Symp Proc.* 7, 27, 2002.
26. Gasparro, F.P. The role of PUVA in the treatment of psoriasis. Photobiology issues related to skin-cancer incidence. *Am J Clin Dermatol.* 1, 337, 2000.
27. Ahmad, M. et al. Identification and characterization of murine caspase-14, a new member of the caspase family. *Cancer Res.* 58, 5201, 1998.
28. Hu, S. et al. Caspase-14 is a novel developmentally regulated protease. *J Biol Chem.* 273, 29648, 1998.
29. Van de Craen, M. et al. Identification of a new caspase homologue: Caspase-14. *Cell Death Differ.* 5, 838, 1998.
30. Eckhart, L. et al. Caspase-14: Analysis of gene structure and mRNA expression during keratinocyte differentiation. *Biochem Biophys Res Commun.* 277, 655, 2000.
31. Fischer, H. et al. Stratum corneum-derived caspase-14 is catalytically active. *FEBS Lett.* 577, 446, 2004.

32. Eckhart, L. et al. Terminal differentiation of human keratinocytes and stratum corneum formation is associated with caspase-14 activation. *J Invest Dermatol.* 115, 1148, 2000.

33. Lippens, S. et al. Epidermal differentiation does not involve the pro apoptotic executioner caspases, but is associated with caspase-14 induction and processing. *Cell Death Differ.* 7, 1218, 2000.

34. Pistritto, G. et al. Expression and transcriptional regulation of caspase-14 in simple and complex epithelia. *Cell Death Differ.* 9, 995, 2002.

35. Lippens, S. et al. Caspase 14 is expressed in the epidermis, the choroid plexus, the retinal pigment epithelium and thymic Hassall's bodies. *Cell Death Differ.* 10, 257, 2003.

36. Alibardi, L. et al. Ultrastructural localization of caspase-14 in human epidermis. *J Histochem Cytochem.* 52, 1561, 2004.

37. Rendl, M. et al. Caspase-14 expression by epidermal keratinocytes is regulated by retinoids in a differentiation-associated manner. *J Invest Dermatol.* 119, 1150, 2002.

38. Krajewska, M. et al. Tumor-associated alterations in caspase-14 expression in epithelial malignancies. *Clin Cancer Res.* 11, 5462, 2005.

39. Eckert, R.L. et al. Opposing action of curcumin and green tea polyphenol in human keratinocytes. *Mol Nutr Food Res.* 50, 123, 2006.

40. Zenz, R. et al. Psoriasis-like skin disease and arthritis caused by inducible epidermal deletion of Jun proteins. *Nature.* 437, 369, 2005.

41. Morita, K. et al. Cutaneous ultrastructural features of the flaky skin (*fsn*) mouse mutation. *J Dermatol.* 22, 385, 1995.

42. Sundberg, J.P. et al. Full-thickness skin grafts from flaky skin mice to nude mice: Maintenance of the psoriasiform phenotype. *J Invest Dermatol.* 102, 781, 1994.

43. Kostovic, K. and Pasic, A. Phototherapy of psoriasis: Review and update. *Acta Dermatovenerol Croat.* 12, 42, 2004.

44. Hsu, S. et al. Green tea polyphenols reduced the psoriasiform lesions and regulate caspase 14 by the mitogen-activated protein kinase pathways. *Experimental Dermatology.* 16(8), 678, 2007.

45. Hsu, S. et al. Expression of caspase 14 reduces tumorigenicity of skin cancer cells. *In Vivo*, 21(2), 279, 2007.

46. Yamamoto, T. et al. Role of EGCG-targeted p57/KIP2 in reducing tumorigenicity of oral carcinoma cells and blocking c-jun N-terminal kinase-mediated apoptosis. *Toxicol. Appl. Pharmacol.* 224, 318, 2007.

CHAPTER 8

Pomegranate Phenolic Antioxidant Activities Protect against Cardiovascular Diseases

Michael Aviram, Mira Rosenblat, and Bianca Fuhrman

CONTENTS

POLYPHENOLIC FLAVONOIDS AND CARDIOVASCULAR DISEASES

Polyphenolic flavonoids compose the largest and the most studied group of plant phenolics. More than 4000 different flavonoids have been identified to date. Flavonoids are grouped into anthocyanins and anthoxantins. Anthocyanins are glycosides

of anthocyanidin, and they are the most important group of water-soluble plant pigments, responsible for the red, blue, and purple colors of flowers and fruits. Anthoxantins are colorless or colored white-to-yellow, and include flavonols, flavanols,
flavones, flavans, and isoflavones. Flavonoids are powerful antioxidants, and their
activity is related to their chemical structure.[1,2] Plant flavonoids can act as potent
inhibitors of low-density lipoprotein (LDL) oxidation[3,4] or of macrophage oxidation.[5]
Dietary consumption of flavonoids was shown to be inversely related to morbidity and mortality from coronary heart disease.[6] Moreover, an inverse association
between flavonoid intake and subsequent occurrence of ischemic heart disease or
cerebrovascular disease was shown.[7,8] Reduced morbidity and mortality from cardiovascular diseases, in spite of high intake of saturated fat among the French—the so-
called "French paradox"[9]—has been attributed to the regular intake of red wine in
the diet. Dietary consumption of flavonoid-rich nutrients, as well as pure flavonoids,
was shown to attenuate the progression of atherosclerosis in animals.[10] Reduced
development of atherosclerotic lesion areas in the atherosclerotic apolipoprotein E
deficient (E[0]) mice was demonstrated following consumption of red wine,[11,12] licorice
root extract,[13,14] grape powder,[15] or ginger extract.[16]

POMEGRANATE JUICE POLYPHENOLS INHIBIT
DEVELOPMENT OF ATHEROSCLEROTIC LESIONS

The pomegranate tree, which is said to have flourished in the Garden of Eden,
has been extensively used as a folk medicine in many cultures.[17,18] Edible parts of
pomegranate fruits (about 50% of total fruit weight) comprise 80% juice and 20%
seeds. Fresh juice contains 85% moisture, 10% total sugars, 1.5% pectin, ascorbic
acid, and polyphenols.

Content of soluble polyphenols in pomegranate juice (PJ) varies within the limits of 0.2–1.0%, depending on the variety, and includes mainly anthocyanins (such
as cyanidin-3-glycoside, cyanidin-3, 3-diglycoside, and delphindin-3-glucoside) and
anthoxantins (such as catechins, ellagic tannins, and gallic and ellagic acids).[19,20]
Ellagic acid and hydrolyzable ellagitannins are both implicated in protection against
atherogenesis, along with their potent antioxidant capacity. Punicalagin is the major
ellagitannin in PJ, and this compound is responsible for the high antioxidant activity of this juice. As a major source for polyphenolics, PJ was shown to be a very
potent antioxidant against LDL oxidation and, in parallel, to inhibit atherosclerosis
development in mice and in humans.[21–23] In vivo studies were conducted first in order
to evaluate whether the active antioxidant components of PJ are absorbed. Recent
studies examined the bioavailability and metabolism of punicalagin in the rat as an
animal model.[24,25]

Two groups of rats were studied. One group was fed with a standard rat diet ($n = 5$)
and the second one with the same diet plus 6% punicalagin ($n = 5$). The daily intake of
punicalagin ranged from 0.6 to 1.2 g. In plasma, glucuronides of methyl ether derivatives of ellagic acid and punicalagin were detected. 6H-Dibenzo[b,d]pyran-6-one
derivatives were also observed in the plasma, especially during the last few weeks of

the study. In urine, the main metabolites observed were the 6H-dibenzo[b,d]pyran-6-one derivatives, which were present as aglycones or as glucuronides. It was concluded that since only 3–6% of the ingested punicalagin was detected as such or as metabolites in urine and feces, the majority of this ellagitannin has to be converted to undetectable metabolites or accumulated in nonanalyzed tissues. Only traces of punicalagin metabolites were detected in liver or kidney.

In humans, following consumption of PJ (180 mL) containing 25 mg of ellagic acid and 318 mg of hydrolyzable ellagitannins (as punicalagin), ellagic acid was detected in human plasma 1 hour after ingestion at a maximum concentration of 32 ng/mL, and by 4 hours it was completely eliminated.[26] Thus, active components of PJ are indeed absorbed, and subsequently affect biological processes, which are related to atherogenesis protection. Upon analyzing the influence of the physiological conditions in the stomach and small intestine on pomegranate bioactive compound bioavailability using an *in vitro* availability method, it was demonstrated that pomegranate phenolic compounds are available during digestion in a high amount (29%). Nevertheless, due to pH, anthocyanins are largely transformed into nonred forms, or degraded.[27]

Studies in Atherosclerotic Mice

PJ supplementation to the atherosclerotic E^0 mice reduced the size of their atherosclerotic lesions and the number of foam cells in their lesions,[28] in comparison to control placebo-treated E^0 mice that were supplemented with water. We also analyzed the therapeutic potency of PJ by its administration to E^0 mice with already advanced atherosclerosis. Atherosclerotic E^0 mice at 4 months of age were supplemented for 2 months with 31 μL of PJ (equivalent to 0.875 μmol of total polyphenols per mouse per day, which is equivalent to about one 8-ounce glass per human per day), and were compared to age-matched placebo-treated mice, as well as to the second control group of 4-month-old mice. Although the atherosclerotic lesion areas in the PJ-treated mice were increased in comparison to the lesion size observed in the control younger mice (4 months of age), PJ supplementation was still able to reduce the mice atherosclerotic lesion size by 17%, in comparison to atherosclerotic lesion of the age-matched placebo-treated mice (Figure 8.1A–C).[29] These results were further confirmed by de Nigris et al.,[30] who demonstrated that oral administration of PJ to hypercholesterolemic LDL-receptor deficient mice at various stages of the disease reduced significantly the progression of atherosclerosis. Thus, PJ exhibits preventive as well as therapeutic effects against atherosclerosis.

Studies in Humans

We next investigated the effects of PJ consumption by patients with carotid artery stenosis (CAS) on carotid lesion size in association with changes in oxidative stress.[31] Ten patients were supplemented with PJ for up to 1 year, and nine CAS patients who did not consume PJ served as a control group. Blood samples were collected before treatment and after 3, 6, 9, and 12 months of PJ consumption. Patients' carotid

The Effect of Pomegranate Juice on Atherosclerotic Lesion Area in E^0-Mice

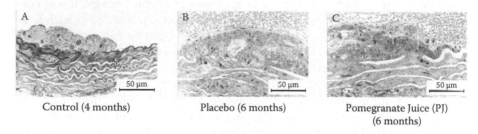

Control (4 months)   Placebo (6 months)   Pomegranate Juice (PJ)
                                                                (6 months)

The Effect of Pomegranate Juice on Carotid Intima Media Thickness (IMT)
and on End Diastolic Velocity (EDV) in Carotid Artery Stenosis (CAS) Patients

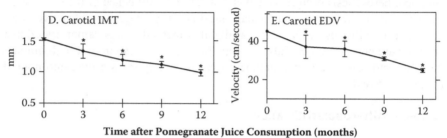

Time after Pomegranate Juice Consumption (months)

Figure 8.1 Therapeutic effect of pomegranate juice on atherosclerotic lesion area in E^0 mice (A–C) or in patients with carotid artery stenosis (D and E). Thirty E^0 mice and 10 patients with severe CAS were supplemented with PJ concentrate (12.5 µL/mouse/day and 50 mL/day, respectively) for 9 weeks or for 1 year, respectively. Photomicrographs of typical foam cells from unsupplemented 4-month-old E^0 mice and from 6-month-old E^0 mice administered a placebo (B) or PJ (C) are presented. Mean (±SEM) effect of PJ consumption on human common carotid artery IMT (D) and end diastolic velocity (EDV) (E) are shown. * = $p < 0.01$ (after vs. before PJ consumption).

intima-media thickness (IMT) was compared between the PJ group and the control group. The ultrasound outcome data were the change over time in maximal IMT, which was measured in the same preselected carotid artery segments. While in the control group (no PJ) IMT increased by 10% after 1 year, PJ consumption resulted in a significant IMT reduction by up to 35% (Figure 8.1D). Analysis of the mean carotid IMT (of the left and right common carotid arteries) before and during PJ consumption revealed a gradual reduction of 13, 22, 26, and 35%, as observed after 3, 6, 9, and 12 months of PJ consumption, respectively, in comparison to baseline values ("0 time," Figure 8.1D). On examination of the internal carotid arteries, flow velocities were calculated at the stenotic sites and expressed by peak systolic velocity (PSV) and end diastolic velocity (EDV). Twelve months of PJ consumption resulted in PSV reduction by 12 and 28% in the left and right carotid arteries, respectively. Mean carotid EDV of both left and right carotid arteries gradually decreased, by 16, 20, 31, and 44% after 3, 6, 9, and 12 months of PJ consumption, respectively (Figure 8.1E). Thus, PJ consumption by patients with CAS decreases atherosclerotic lesion size, and these effects could be related to the potent antioxidant characteristics of PJ.

ANTIOXIDATIVE PROPERTIES OF POMEGRANATE JUICE

Antioxidative Capacity of Pomegranate Juice in Comparison to Other Juices

Pomegranate juice was shown to possess an antioxidant activity that was three times higher than the antioxidant activity of green tea.[19] The antioxidant activity was higher in juice extracted from whole pomegranate than in juice obtained from arils only, suggesting that the processing extracts some of the hydrolyzable tannins present in the fruit rind into the juice.

We have demonstrated that pomegranate juice contains a higher concentration of total polyphenols (5 mmol/L) in comparison to other fruit juices (orange, grapefruit, grape, cranberry, pear, pineapple, apple, and peach juices, which contain only 1.3–4 mmol/L of total polyphenols; Figure 8.2A). A similar pattern was noted for the IC_{50} values obtained for the inhibition of copper ion-induced LDL oxidation. While PJ exhibited a very low IC_{50} (0.06 μL/mL), the IC_{50} values for the other juices were in the range of 0.11–7.50 μL/mL (Figure 8.2B). The most potent antioxidant activity of PJ could be related to its high polyphenolic flavonoid content, as well as to the specific type of potent polyphenols present in PJ (specific hydrolyzable tannins).

Contribution of Pomegranate Juice Constituents to Its Antioxidative Properties

Several polyphenolic fractions were isolated from pomegranate juice, including gallic acid, ellagic acid, tannins, total PJ anthocyanins, and specific anthocyanins, such as cyanidin-3-0-β-glucopyranoside, cyanidin-3,5-di-0-β-glucopyranoside, delphinidin-3-0-β-glucopyranoside, and pelargenin-3-0-β-glucopyranoside. The total anthocyanin and tannin fractions exhibited a dose-dependent antioxidative effect against copper ion–induced LDL oxidation. In the 2,2 azobis 2-amidino propane hydrochloride (AAPH)-induced LDL oxidation process, both fractions exhibited weaker antioxidative properties in comparison to the copper ion–induced LDL oxidation. These results suggest that the anthocyanins and tannins possess, in addition to their free radical scavenging capabilities, transition metal ion chelation properties. The tannin fraction was more potent than the anthocyanin fraction in inhibiting LDL oxidation, and the IC_{50} of the tannins was half that of the anthocyanins. Both PJ ellagic and gallic acids and the anthocyanins delphinidin-3-0-β-glucopyranoside, pelargonidin-3-0-β-glucopyranoside, cyanidin-3-0-β-glucopyranoside, and cyanidin-3,5-di-0-β-glucopyranoside inhibited copper ion–induced LDL oxidation in a dose-dependent manner.

Upon comparing the effects of ellagic acid to gallic acid, gallic acid was a more potent inhibitor of LDL oxidation (IC_{50} of 2.1 μg/mL for gallic acid vs. 16 μg/mL for ellagic acid). Similarly, the anthocyanins delphinidin-3-0-β-glucopyranoside and cyanidin-3-0-β-glucopyranoside were more potent antioxidants against LDL oxidation than ellagic acid, with IC_{50} of 3.0, 2.0, and 16 μg/mL, respectively. When comparing the antioxidative properties of the specific PJ anthocyanins, pelargonidin-

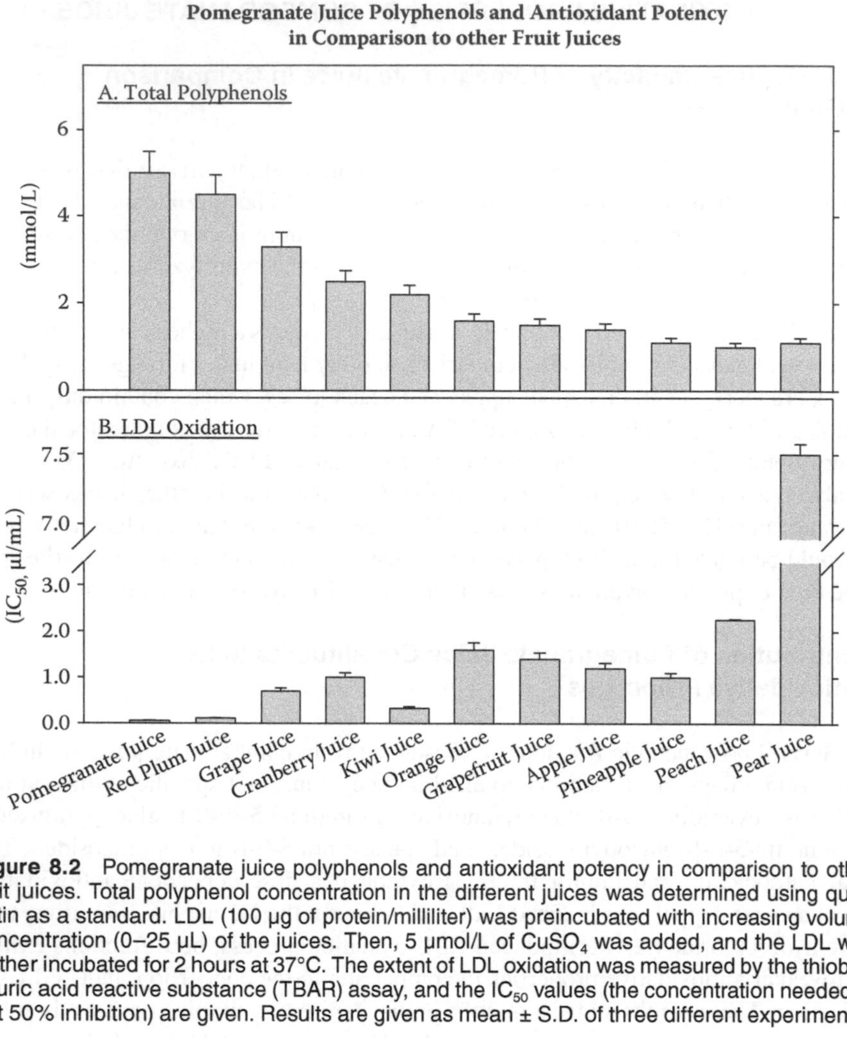

Pomegranate Juice Polyphenols and Antioxidant Potency
in Comparison to other Fruit Juices

Figure 8.2 Pomegranate juice polyphenols and antioxidant potency in comparison to other fruit juices. Total polyphenol concentration in the different juices was determined using quercetin as a standard. LDL (100 µg of protein/milliliter) was preincubated with increasing volume concentration (0–25 µL) of the juices. Then, 5 µmol/L of $CuSO_4$ was added, and the LDL was further incubated for 2 hours at 37°C. The extent of LDL oxidation was measured by the thiobarbituric acid reactive substance (TBAR) assay, and the IC_{50} values (the concentration needed to get 50% inhibition) are given. Results are given as mean ± S.D. of three different experiments.

3-0-β-glucopyranoside and cyanidin-3,5-di-0-β-glucopyranoside were less potent than delphinidin-3-0-β-glucopyranoside or cyanidin-3-0-β-glucopyranoside (IC_{50} of 13 µg/mL vs. 2–3 µg/mL). A similar pattern was noted for the free radical scavenging capabilities of the preceding PJ fractions.

POMEGRANATE JUICE CONSUMPTION
REDUCES SERUM OXIDATIVE STRESS

Serum Lipid Peroxidation

Human plasma obtained from healthy men after 2 weeks of PJ consumption (50 mL PJ concentrate/day, equivalent to 1.5 mmol total polyphenols) demonstrated a

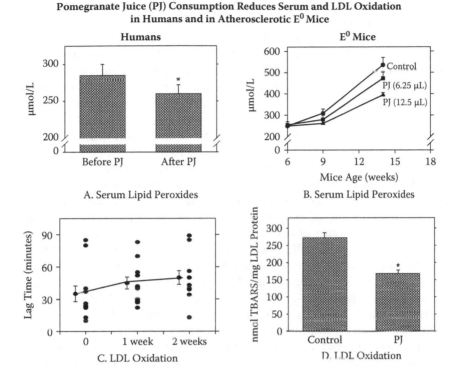

Pomegranate Juice (PJ) Consumption Reduces Serum and LDL Oxidation in Humans and in Atherosclerotic E^0 Mice

A. Serum Lipid Peroxides

B. Serum Lipid Peroxides

C. LDL Oxidation

D. LDL Oxidation

Figure 8.3 Pomegranate juice consumption reduces serum and LDL oxidation in humans and in atherosclerotic E^0 mice. Mean (±SD) effect of 2 and 9 weeks of PJ supplementation to 13 healthy men and to E^0 mice (A and B, respectively) on the susceptibility of serum to radical-induced lipid peroxidation and copper ion–induced LDL oxidation (C and D, respectively) is shown. * = $p < 0.01$ (after vs. before PJ consumption in humans, and PJ vs. control in mice).

small but significant ($p < 0.01$) 16% decreased susceptibility to free radical–induced lipid peroxidation, in comparison to plasma obtained prior to PJ consumption, as measured by lipid peroxide formation (Figure 8.3A) or as total antioxidant status (TAS) in serum. To determine the effect of increasing or decreasing the dosages of PJ on plasma lipid peroxidation, and to analyze PJ capability to maintain its effect after termination of juice consumption, three subjects were further studied. Supplementation of 20 mL of PJ concentrate/day for 1 week resulted in a significant decrease of 11% in plasma lipid peroxidation, compared to plasma obtained prior to PJ consumption. Supplementation of 50 mL PJ concentrate/day for 1 more week exhibited a further 21% decrease in plasma lipid peroxidation. However, a further increase in the supplemented PJ to 80 mL of PJ concentrate/day for an additional week did not further inhibit plasma susceptibility to lipid peroxidation.

Gradual decreasing of the PJ dosage in these three subjects down to 40 mL/day for 1 week, and then to 20 mL/day for an additional 2 weeks, did not significantly affect plasma lipid peroxidation, which remained low in comparison to the levels obtained after supplementation of 80 mL of PJ concentrate/day. Two weeks after cessation of PJ supplementation, the reduced rate of plasma susceptibility to lipid peroxidation, was sustained. After a further 4 weeks with no PJ consumption, plasma lipid peroxidation returned to the higher values obtained before PJ consumption.

The effect of PJ consumption by patients with CAS on their serum oxidative state was measured also as serum concentration of antibodies against Ox-LDL.[31] A significant ($p < 0.01$) reduction in the concentration of antibodies against Ox-LDL by 24 and 19% was observed after 1 and 3 months of PJ consumption, respectively (from 2070 ± 61 EU/mL before treatment to 1563 ± 69 and 1670 ± 52 EU/mL after 1 and 3 months of PJ consumption, respectively). Total antioxidant status (TAS) in serum from these patients was substantially increased by 2.3-fold (from 0.95 ± 0.12 nmol/L at baseline up to 2.20 ± 0.25 nmol/L after 12 months of PJ consumption). These results indicate that PJ administration to patients with CAS substantially reduced their serum oxidative status and could thus inhibit plasma lipid peroxidation. The susceptibility of the patient's plasma to free radical–induced oxidation decreased after 12 months of PJ consumption by 62% (from 209 ± 18 at baseline to 79 ± 6 nmol of peroxides/milliliter). The effect of PJ consumption on serum oxidative state was recently measured also in patients with non-insulin-dependent diabetes mellitus (NIDDM). Consumption of 50 mL of PJ per day for a period of 3 months resulted in a significant reduction in serum lipid peroxides and thiobarbituric acid reactive substance (TBAR) levels by 56 and 28%, respectively.[32]

PJ consumption exhibited antioxidative effects also when administered to E^0 mice.[28] The basal oxidative state, measured as lipid peroxides in plasma of control E^0 mice (that did not consume PJ), increased gradually during aging from 260 nmol/mL of plasma at 6 weeks of age to 309 and 535 nmol/mL of plasma after 9 and 14 weeks of age, respectively. Following PJ consumption, plasma lipid peroxidation was markedly reduced, and this effect was PJ concentration dependent (Figure 8.3B). Similarly, serum total antioxidant status was higher in E^0 mice that consumed PJ in comparison to control mice, and this effect was again juice concentration dependent.[28]

Pomegranate peel extracts have also been shown to possess significant antioxidant activity. Albino rats of the Wistar strain were fed a dried methanolic extract from pomegranate peels at 50 mg/kg (in terms of catechin equivalents) followed by carbon tetrachloride (CCl_4)-induced oxidative stress. This resulted in preservation of catalase, peroxidase, and superoxide dismutase (SOD) activity to values comparable with control values, whereas lipid peroxidation was brought back by 54% as compared to control.[33]

LDL and HDL Oxidation

Consumption of PJ for 1 and 2 weeks by healthy volunteers increased the resistance of their LDL to copper ion–induced oxidation, as shown by a prolongation of the lag time required for the initiation of LDL oxidation, by 29 and 43%, in comparison to LDL obtained prior to juice consumption (Figure 8.3C).[28] Similarly, the resistance of their high-density lipoprotein (HDL) to copper ion–induced oxidation also gradually increased after PJ consumption, as shown by a prolongation in the lag time required for the initiation of HDL oxidation from 37 ± 2 minutes to 45 ± 6 minutes before and 2 weeks after PJ consumption, respectively. PJ consumption by patients with CAS resulted in a significant reduction in the basal level of LDL-associated lipid peroxides by 43, 89, 86, and 90% after 3, 6, 9, and 12 months of PJ consumption, respectively, and in parallel it increased the resistance of LDL to copper ion–induced oxidation.[31]

This was demonstrated by reduced formation of lipid peroxides in LDL during its incubation with copper ions (by 40, 49, 57, and 59% after 3, 6, 9, and 12 months of PJ consumption, respectively). PJ consumption also decreased the propensity of LDL derived from E^0 mice to copper ion–induced oxidation (Figure 8.3D). In E^0 mice that consumed 6.25 or 12.5 μL/day of PJ concentrate for a period of 2 months, LDL oxidation was delayed by 100 and 120 minutes, respectively, in comparison to LDL obtained before juice administration. Determination of the extent of LDL oxidation by the TBAR assay revealed a significant inhibition after PJ consumption (Figure 8.3D). Furthermore, the progressive increase with age in the susceptibility of the mice LDL to oxidation was significantly attenuated by PJ consumption in a dose-dependent manner.[28]

Paraoxonase 1 (PON1)

The increased resistance of LDL and of HDL to oxidation after PJ administration to healthy subjects or to patients with CAS could have also resulted from increased serum HDL–associated paraoxonase activity. Indeed, a significant 18% increase in serum paraoxonase (PON 1) activity was monitored in healthy subjects after PJ consumption for a period of 2 weeks.[28] In CAS patients, serum paraoxonase 1 (measured as arylesterase activity) significantly increased by 11, 42, 49, and 83% after 3, 6, 9, and 12 months of PJ consumption, respectively[31]; in NIDDM patients it significantly increased by 12% after PJ consumption for 3 months.[32] Similar to the results obtained in humans, a significant 43% increase in serum paraoxonase activity was also observed in E^0 mice after PJ consumption for a period of 2 months, in comparison to serum paraoxonase activity observed in the placebo-treated mice.[29] The increase in serum paraoxonase activity may be a direct effect of PJ, as well as an effect secondary to PJ-mediated reduction in lipid peroxides. It was previously demonstrated that paraoxonase is inactivated by oxidized lipids,[34] and its activity is preserved by antioxidants, including the red wine flavonoids or the licorice-derived isoflavan glabridin. PJ contains very potent antioxidants and, unlike other nutrients,[34] it not only preserves serum PON1, but also increases the enzyme activity.

POMEGRANATE JUICE REDUCES MACROPHAGE
ATHEROGENICITY *IN VIVO* AND *IN VITRO*

Oxidative stress, which has been implicated in the pathogenesis of atherosclerosis,[35,36] has been shown to considerably attack lipids, not only in LDL, but also in arterial macrophages.[37,38] We have previously shown that "lipid-peroxidized macrophages" exhibit atherogenic characteristics, including increased ability to oxidize LDL and to take up oxidized LDL (Ox-LDL).[39]

LDL oxidation by macrophages is considered to be the hallmark of early atherogenesis, and it is associated with cellular uptake of oxidatively modified LDL, leading to macrophage cholesterol accumulation and foam cell formation. We thus studied the effect of dietary consumption of PJ by E^0 mice on macrophage atherogenicity, including macrophage lipid peroxidation and subsequently macrophage activities related to foam cell formation, such as cell-mediated oxidation of LDL and cellular uptake of lipoproteins.

Macrophage Oxidative Stress

We have demonstrated that human monocyte derived macrophages (HMDMs) isolated from NIDDM patients after consumption of PJ for 3 months, the carotid lesion derived after endartherectomy from CAS patients that consumed PJ (Figure 8.4A), and also mouse peritoneal macrophages (MPMs) isolated from E^0 mice after consumption of PJ concentrate (12.5 μL/mouse/day, equivalent to 0.35 μmol of total

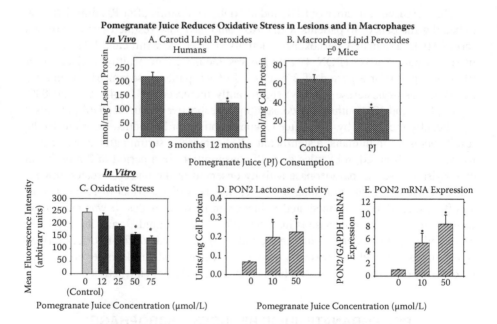

Figure 8.4 Pomegranate juice reduces oxidative stress in lesions and in macrophages: *in vivo* and *in vitro* studies. Mean (±SD) of the effect of PJ consumption on lipid peroxides in human carotid lesions (A) and in mouse peritoneal macrophages (B). J774 A1 macrophages were incubated with increasing concentrations of PJ for 90 minutes at 37°C. (C) Cellular oxidative stress measured as DCFH oxidation, (D) PON2 lactonase activity, and (E) PON2 mRNA expression. * = p < 0.01 (after vs. before PJ consumption in humans, and PJ vs. control in mice, and incubation *in vitro* with PJ vs. control without PJ).

polyphenols) for a period of 2 months (Figure 8.4B) contained less lipid peroxide, in comparison to carotid lesion from patients that did not consume PJ, or to MPMs from control E^0 mice, respectively.[28,32] Incubation of the human carotid lesion or of E^0 mouse peritoneal macrophages with LDL (100 µg of protein/milliliter) for 18 hours under oxidative stress (in the presence of copper ions) revealed that PJ consumption resulted in 43 and 82% reduced capacity of the lesion or the macrophages to oxidize LDL, respectively. The mechanism responsible for this effect was associated with inhibition of the translocation to the macrophage plasma membrane of the nicotin-amide adenine dinucleotide phosphate (NADPH) oxidase cytosolic factor p-47, and, hence, inhibition of NADPH oxidase activation. As a result of this, a reduction (by 49%) in superoxide anion release from the macrophages and an elevation in cellular glutathione content, by 25%, were observed. These effects could also be related to the decreased levels of macrophage-associated lipid peroxides after PJ consump-tion, in comparison to macrophages isolated from control E^0 mice that consumed placebo.

On a molecular basis, PJ could interfere with macrophage oxidative status and macrophage-mediated LDL oxidation by affecting redox-sensitive gene transcrip-tion. The activation of nuclear factor κ-B (NFκ-B), the oxidative stress responsive transcription factor, has been linked with a variety of inflammatory diseases, including atherosclerosis. Extensive research in the last few years, reviewed by Aggarwal and Shishoda,[40] has shown that the pathway that activates NFκ-B can be inhibited by phytochemicals, including those present in pomegranate, and thus provide a beneficial effect against atherosclerosis development. It was demonstrated that pomegranate wine (PJ fermented with yeast and dealcoholized) inhibits oxida-tion of endothelial cells induced by tumor necrosis factor (TNF)-α, and acts as a potent inhibitor of NFκ-B activation in these cells.[41] Pomegranate fermented juice and pomegranate cold-pressed seed oil flavonoids were also shown to inhibit eico-sanoid enzyme activity.[42] Flavonoids extracted from pomegranate cold-pressed seed oil showed 31–44% inhibition of sheep cyclooxygenase and 69–81% inhibition of soybean lipoxygenase. Flavonoids extracted from pomegranate fermented juice also showed 21–30% inhibition of soybean lipoxygenase. Recently, it was demonstrated that PJ decreased the activation of the redox-sensitive genes ELK-1 and p-JUN and increased eNOS expression in cultured endothelial cells exposed to shear stress, as well as in atherosclerotic-prone areas of hypercholesterolemic mice.[30]

The PJ-mediated reduction in the transcription of several key redox enzymes, including cyclooxygenase, lipoxygenase, and NO synthase, could be the result of intracellular oxidation suppression. Through this mechanism, as well as via the sup-pression of lipoxygenase-catalyzed leukotriene formation, PJ may act also as an anti-inflammatory agent, in addition to its major role as antioxidant.

Macrophage Cholesterol Metabolism

Macrophage cholesterol accumulation and foam cell formation are the hallmark of early atherogenesis. Cholesterol accumulation in macrophages can result from impaired balance between external and internal cholesterol sources. LDL, which undergoes oxidative modification, is an important external source for macrophage accumulated cholesterol.

Ox-LDL is taken up by macrophages at an enhanced rate via scavenger receptors,[43,44] which, unlike the LDL receptor, are not down-regulated by intracellular cholesterol content[45] and therefore lead to accumulation of cholesterol in the cells. Macrophage cholesterol from internal sources originates from the cholesterol biosynthesis. The enzyme 3-hydroxy-3 methylglutaryl coenzyme A (HMGCoA) reductase catalyzes the rate-limiting step in the cholesterol biosynthetic pathway,[46] and it is subjected to a negative feedback regulation by the cellular cholesterol content. In addition to cellular uptake of lipoproteins and to cholesterol biosynthesis, macrophage cholesterol accumulation can also result from a decreased efflux of cholesterol from the cells.[47]

Since PJ was shown to inhibit macrophage foam cell formation and the development of atherosclerotic lesions, we analyzed the effect of PJ consumption on cellular processes that lead to macrophage cholesterol accumulation. We have demonstrated that the cellular uptake of Ox-LDL, measured as cellular lipoprotein binding, cell association, and degradation, by MPMs derived from E^0 mice that consumed 12.5 μL of PJ concentrate/mouse/day for a period of 2 months was significantly reduced (by 16, 22, and 15%, respectively) in comparison to Ox-LDL binding, cell association, and degradation obtained by MPMs from control E^0 mice. Similarly, PJ consumption by NIDDM patients significantly decreased the extent of Ox-LDL cellular uptake by their HMDM (by 36%).[32] Cellular cholesterol esterification rate (another atherogenic property of macrophages) in MPMs isolated from PJ-treated mice was found to be 80% lower compared with age-matched, placebo-treated mice. Finally, PJ treatment significantly increased, by 39%, cholesterol efflux from macrophages compared with the cholesterol efflux rate from MPMs harvested from the placebo-treated mice. Taken together, all these anti-atherogenic effects lead to reduced accumulation of cholesterol in macrophages.

In vitro studies clearly show that PJ exhibits direct anti-atherogenic effects on macrophages. Pre-incubation of macrophages in culture (J774A.1 cell line) with PJ resulted in a significant ($p < 0.01$) reduction in Ox-LDL degradation by 40%.[48] On the other hand, PJ had no effect on macrophage degradation of native LDL or on macrophage cholesterol efflux. Macrophage cholesterol biosynthesis, however, was inhibited by 50% after cell incubation with PJ. This inhibition, unlike statin action, was not mediated by an effect on HMGCoA reductase along the cholesterol biosynthetic pathway. In addition, pre-incubation of J774A.1 macrophages with increasing concentrations of PJ dose-dependently reduced macrophage oxidative stress (Figure 8.4C). Recently, we have demonstrated that unique complex sugars and/or phenolics in PJ also contribute to PJ-induced reduction of macrophage oxidative stress.[49] Increasing concentrations of the PJ sugar fractions resulted in a dose-dependent decrement in macrophage (J774 A.1) peroxide levels compared to control cells—up to 72%. In contrast, incubation of the cells with white grape juice sugar fraction at the same concentration resulted in a dose-dependent increment in peroxide levels up to 37%.

Furthermore, we have recently demonstrated that PJ and phenolics derived from PJ (punicalagin and gallic acid) up-regulate the enzyme paraoxonase 2 (PON2) lactonase activity (Figure 8.4D), mRNA (Figure 8.4E), and protein expression in macrophages. PON2 is a member of the paraoxonase gene family, and similarly to the antioxidative effect of the humoral PON1 in serum, PON2 was shown to protect macrophages against oxidative stress. Thus, the antioxidative characteristics of PJ unique phenolics punicalagin and gallic acid could be related, at least in part, to their stimulatory effect on macrophage PON2 expression. This phenomenon was shown to be associated with PJ-mediated activation of the transcription factors PAPRγ and AP-1.[50]

We conclude that PJ protects the macrophages against oxidative stress by increasing PON2 expression, suppressing Ox-LDL uptake by macrophages, and inhibiting cellular cholesterol biosynthesis, leading to attenuation in cellular cholesterol accumulation and foam cell formation.

ANTI-ATHEROGENIC EFFECTS OF POMEGRANATE BY-PRODUCTS

A product of total pomegranate tannins (TPT) containing 85% punicalagin, 1.3% ellagic acid, and a small amount of ellagic acid glycosides was purified from the pomegranate husk extract prepared by Dr. Navindra P. Seeram from the laboratory of Dr. David Heber at the University of California, Los Angeles (UCLA), California.[51] On a similar polyphenol weight basis (10 μg/mL), TPT was more potent than vitamin E or PJ when analyzed as a free radical scavenger. TPT reduces the absorbance in the DPPH solution by 75% in comparison to 62 and 48% reduction obtained by a similar total polyphenol content of PJ or vitamin E, respectively. LDL oxidation induced either by copper ions or AAPH was dose-dependently inhibited by TPT, with an IC_{50} of 2.1 and 1.4 μg/mL, respectively. Macrophage oxidative status was also substantially decreased by 50% on using 80 μmol/mL of TPT polyphenols. At a similar concentration, punicalagin was found to be even more potent than TPT in all the preceding assays.

The antioxidative properties of pomegranate polyphenol extract powder as well as of pomegranate fiber powder were also analyzed. The pomegranate fiber powder polyphenol concentration was eightfold lower, as compared to the polyphenols in the pomegranate extract powder (200 ± 6 nmol/mg vs. 1580 ± 138 nmol/mg, respectively). The pomegranate extract was significantly more potent than the fiber powder in both scavenging of free radicals and in reducing macrophage oxidative stress.

The effects of a pomegranate liquid by-product (PBP), which includes the whole pomegranate fruit left over after juice preparation, on atherosclerosis development in apolipoprotein E-deficient (E^0) mice were studied.[52] Consumption of PBP (17 or 51.5 mg gallic acid equivalents/kilogram/day) by the mice resulted in a significant reduction in atherosclerotic lesion size by up to 57% (Figure 8.5A). PBP consumption significantly reduced oxidative stress in the MPMs: Cellular lipid peroxide content decreased by up to 42% (Figure 8.5B), and paraoxonase 2 lactonase activity

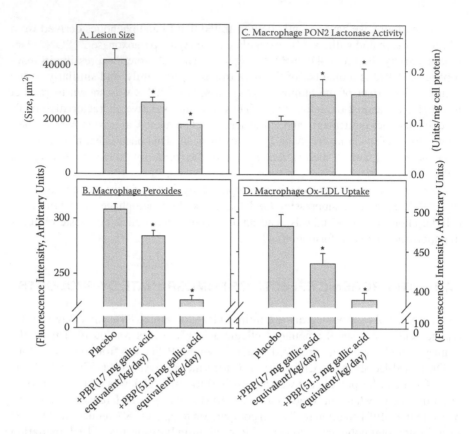

Figure 8.5 Pomegranate by-product (PBP) consumption by E⁰ mice attenuates atherosclerotic lesion development, in association with reduction in macrophage oxidative stress and Ox-LDL uptake. E⁰ mice consumed PBP (17 or 51.5 mg gallic acid equivalents/kilogram/day) for 3 months. Control mice received only water (placebo). At the end of the study, the mice aortas as well as the mice peritoneal macrophages were harvested. (A) Atherosclerotic lesion size determination. (B) Total macrophage peroxide levels were determined by the DCFH-DH assay. (C) For determination of macrophage paraoxonase 2 (PON2) lactonase activity, cells (2 × 10⁶) were incubated with 1 mmol/L dihydrocoumarin in Tris buffer, and the hydrolysis rate was determined after 10 min of incubation at 25°C. (D) The extent of Ox-LDL (25 µg of protein/milliliter, labeled with FITC) uptake by the mice macrophages (1 × 10⁶) was determined by flow cytometry. Results are expressed as mean ±S.D. of three different determinations. * = p < 0.01 versus placebo.

increased by up to 50% (Figure 8.5C), as compared to MPMs from E⁰ mice that consumed only water. Furthermore, oxidized LDL (Ox-LDL) uptake by the MPMs was reduced by up to 19% (Figure 8.5D). Similar results were observed also *in vitro*. Treatment of J774 A.1 macrophages with PBP (10 or 50 µmol/L of total polyphenols) significantly decreased both cellular total peroxide content and Ox-LDL uptake. We thus conclude that PBP significantly attenuates atherosclerosis development by its antioxidant properties.

Next, we performed *ex vivo* and *in vitro* studies in which we compared the antiatherogenic properties of whole pomegranate fruit powder by-product (POMxp) to those of arils + seeds powder. Per milligram of powder, the POMxp contained 90-fold higher concentrations of polyphenols than the arils + seeds. Administration of 10 mg total polyphenols/kilogram/day of POMxp or of arils + seeds aqueous extract to E^0 mice for 2 months demonstrated that POMxp polyphenols are more potent than aril + seed polyphenols in reducing oxidative stress. The amount of superoxide anion released from the MPMs derived from E^0 mice that consumed POMxp or arils + seeds was lower by 39 or 14%, respectively, as compared to the amount released by MPM harvested from the control mice, which received only water (placebo). The extent of Ox-LDL uptake by MPM from mice that consumed POMxp, but not by MPM from the mice that consumed arils + seeds, was significantly reduced by 13%, as compared to Ox-LDL uptake by the control mice MPMs (Figure 8.6A).

Furthermore, consumption of POMxp or of arils + seeds by the E^0 mice significantly stimulated HDL-mediated cholesterol efflux from the mice MPM by 74 and 31%, respectively (Figure 8.6B), indicating that the polyphenols in POMxp are more potent than the polyphenols in the by-product prepared from the arils + seeds in attenuation of macrophage cholesterol accumulation and foam cell formation. Similar results were observed *in vitro* upon adding POMxp or arils + seeds (10 mg gallic acid equivalents/milliliter) to J774 A.1 macrophages, with 53 or 27% reduction in Ox-LDL uptake by the cells, respectively (Figure 8.6C). Upon adding 41 μg of gallic acid equivalents/milliliter of POMxp or arils + seeds to the cells, HDL-mediated cholesterol efflux was significantly stimulated by 147 and 52%, respectively (Figure 8.6D).

We conclude that pomegranate by-products contain potent polyphenols, which are able to reduce oxidative stress and attenuate macrophage cholesterol accumulation by inhibiting Ox-LDL uptake and stimulating HDL-mediated cholesterol efflux.

PERSPECTIVES AND FUTURE DIRECTIONS

Our current view on the major pathways by which pomegranate polyphenols and pomegranate by-products reduce macrophage foam cell formation and the development of advanced atherosclerosis is summarized in Figure 8.7. Pomegranate polyphenols (either in PJ or in the pomegranate by-products) can protect LDL against cell-mediated oxidation via at least two pathways, including a direct interaction of the polyphenols with the lipoprotein and/or an indirect effect through polyphenol accumulation in arterial macrophages. Pomegranate polyphenols were shown to reduce the capacity of macrophages to oxidize LDL, to directly inhibit LDL oxidation by scavenging reactive oxygen species (ROS) and reactive nitrogen species (RNS), and also indirectly by reducing macrophage capacity to oxidize LDL due to polyphenol accumulation in arterial macrophages. Furthermore, pomegranate polyphenols increase serum paraoxonase 1 activity, resulting in the hydrolysis of lipid peroxides in oxidized lipoproteins and in atherosclerotic lesion. Moreover, PJ has a remarkable effect on the atherogenicity of macrophages. PJ was demonstrated to reduce accumulation of cholesterol in these cells due to inhibition of cellular cholesterol biosynthesis and cellular uptake of oxidized LDL (Ox-LDL). PJ also reduced

150 MICHAEL AVIRAM, MIRA ROSENBLAT, AND BIANCA FUHRMAN

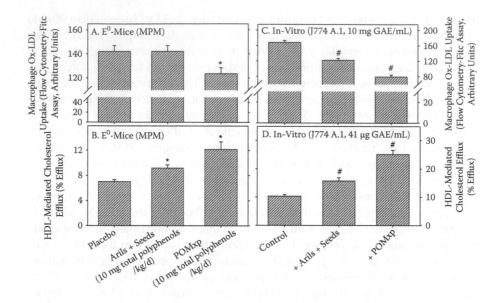

Figure 8.6 Whole pomegranate by-product (POMxp) is more potent than pomegranate by-product arils + seeds in reducing Ox-LDL uptake and in stimulating HDL-mediated macrophage cholesterol efflux. For 2 months, E^0 mice (6 weeks old) consumed 10 mg total polyphenols/kilogram/day of whole pomegranate by-product powder (POMxp) dissolved in water, or of pomegranate by-product arils + seeds liquid extract. Control mice received only water (placebo). At the end of the study, the mice peritoneal macrophages were harvested. (A) The extent of Ox-LDL (25 µg of protein/milliliter, labeled with FITC) uptake by the mice macrophages (1×10^6) was determined by flow cytometry. (B) The mice macrophages were prelabeled with [^{3}H]-cholesterol for 1 hour. Then the cells were washed and further incubated for 3 hours at 37°C without or with HDL (100 µg of protein/milliliter). The extent of HDL-mediated cholesterol efflux was then determined. (C) J774 A.1 macrophages (1×10^6) were incubated for 20 hours at 37°C without (control) or with 10 mg gallic acid equivalents/milliliter of POMxp or of arils + seeds. Then the extent of Ox-LDL uptake was determined as described in B. (D) J774 A.1 macrophages (1×10^6) were incubated for 20 hours at 37°C without (control) or with 41 µg gallic acid equivalents/milliliter of POMxp or of arils + seeds. The extent of HDL-mediated cholesterol efflux from the cells was determined as described in D. Results are given as mean ± S.D of three different determinations. * = p < 0.01 versus placebo; # = p < 0.01 versus control.

the cellular oxidative stress through its stimulatory effect on PON2 expression and consequently a reduction in the oxidative capacity of the cells towards LDL. The pomegranate by-products were similarly shown (both *ex vivo* and *in vitro*) to reduce macrophage oxidative stress and to attenuate macrophage cholesterol accumulation by inhibiting Ox-LDL uptake and by stimulating HDL-mediated cholesterol efflux from the cells.

All these antioxidative and anti-atherogenic effects of pomegranate polyphenols were clearly demonstrated *in vitro*, as well as *in vivo* in humans, and in the atherosclerotic apolipoprotein E–deficient mice. Dietary supplementation of pomegranate juice rich in polyphenols to patients with severe carotid artery stenosis or to atherosclerotic mice resulted in a significant inhibition in the development of the

Pomegranate Attenuates Atherosclerotic Lesion Formation

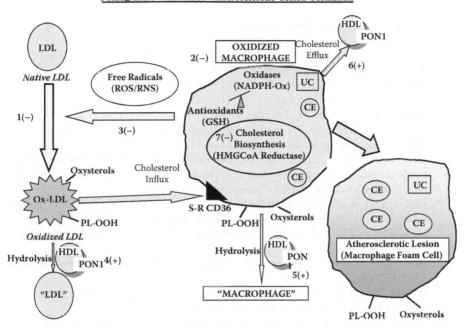

Figure 8.7 Major pathways by which pomegranate polyphenols inhibit macrophage foam cell formation and atherosclerosis. PJ polyphenols affect LDL directly by their interaction with the lipoprotein and inhibition of LDL oxidation (1). PJ polyphenols can also protect LDL indirectly, by their accumulation in arterial cells and protection of arterial macrophages against oxidative stress (2). This latter effect is associated with inhibition of the formation of "oxidized macrophages" via an increase in PON2 expression, and reduction in the capacity of macrophages to oxidize LDL (3). In addition, PJ polyphenols preserve or even increase paraoxonase activity, thereby increasing hydrolysis of lipid peroxides in Ox-LDL (4), in oxidized macrophages in atherosclerotic lesions (5), or increasing HDL-mediated efflux from macrophages (6), leading to attenuation in the progression of atherosclerosis. Furthermore, PJ inhibits cholesterol biosynthesis in macrophages (7), thus reducing cholesterol accumulation in macrophages and their conversion into foam cells. ROS, reactive oxygen species; RNS, reactive nitrogen species; PL-OOH, phospholipid hydroperoxides; S-R, scavenger receptors; CE, cholesterol ester; UC, unesterified cholesterol; (+), stimulation; (−), inhibition.

atherosclerotic lesions, and this may be attributed to the protection of lipids in arterial wall as well as in serum LDL against oxidation. Since combination of antioxidants that exist in PJ and in pomegranate by-product can provide a wider range of free radicals scavenging than an individual antioxidant, clinical and nutritional studies in humans should be directed toward the use of combinations of several types of dietary antioxidants, including combinations of flavonoids together with other nutritional antioxidants, such as vitamin E and carotenoids. It is also important to use reliable biological markers of oxidative stress, and to identify populations suitable for antioxidant treatment, as antioxidant treatment may be beneficial only in subjects under oxidative stress.

REFERENCES

1. Rice-Evans, C.A. et al., The relative antioxidant activities of plant-derived polyphenolic flavonoids, *Free Radic. Res.*, 22, 375, 1995.
2. Van Acker, S.A.B.E. et al., Structural aspects of antioxidants activity of flavonoids, *Free Radic. Biol. Med.*, 20, 331, 1996.
3. Fuhrman, B., and Aviram, M., Flavonoids protect LDL from oxidation and attenuate atherosclerosis, *Curr. Opin. Lipidol.,* 12, 41, 2001.
4. Fuhrman, B., and Aviram, M., Polyphenols and flavonoids protect LDL against atherogenic modifications, in *Handbook of antioxidants: Biochemical, nutritional and clinical aspects,* 2nd ed., Cadenas E., and Packer, L. (eds.), Marcel Dekker, New York, 16, 303, 2001.
5. Rosenblat, M. et al., Macrophage enrichment with the isoflavan glabridin inhibits NADPH oxidase-induced cell-mediated oxidation of low density lipoprotein: A possible role for protein kinase C, *J. Biol. Chem.*, 274, 13790, 1999.
6. Hertog, M.G. et al., Flavonoid intake and long-term risk of coronary heart disease and cancer in the seven countries study, *Arch. Intern. Med.,* 155, 381, 1995.
7. Knekt, P. et al., Flavonoid intake and risk of chronic diseases, *Am. J. Clin. Nutr.*, 76, 560, 2002.
8. Knekt, P. et al., Flavonoid intake and coronary mortality in Finland: A cohort study, *BMJ,* 312, 478, 1996.
9. Renaud, S., and de Lorgeril, M., Wine alcohol, platelets and the French paradox for coronary heart disease, *Lancet,* 339, 1523, 1992.
10. Aviram, M., Antioxidants in restenosis and atherosclerosis, *Curr. Interven. Cardiol. Rep.,* 1, 66, 1999.
11. Hayek, T. et al., Reduced progression of atherosclerosis in the apolipoprotein E-deficient mice following consumption of red wine, or its polyphenols quercetin, or catechin, is associated with reduced susceptibility of LDL to oxidation and aggregation, *Arterioscler. Thromb. Vasc. Biol.*, 17, 2744, 1997.
12. Aviram, M., and Fuhrman, B., Wine flavonoids, LDL cholesterol oxidation and atherosclerosis, in *Wine: A scientific exploration,* Sandler, M. and Pinder, R.M. (eds.), Taylor & Francis, London, 140, 2003.
13. Fuhrman, B. et al., Licorice extract and its major polyphenol glabridin protect low density lipoprotein against lipid peroxidation: *In vitro* and *ex vivo* studies in humans and in atherosclerotic apolipoprotein E-deficient mice, *Am. J. Clin. Nutr.,* 66, 267, 1997.
14. Aviram, M., Vaya, J., and Fuhrman, B., Licorice root flavonoid antioxidants reduce LDL oxidation and attenuate cardiovascular diseases, in *Herbal medicines: Molecular basis of biological activity and health,* Packer L., Halliwel B., and Nam Ong, C. (eds.), Marcel Dekker, New York, 27, 595, 2004.
15. Fuhrman, B. et al., Grape powder polyphenols attenuate atherosclerosis development in apolipoprotein E-deficient (E^0) mice and reduce macrophage atherogenicity, *J. Nutr.,* 135, 722, 2005.
16. Fuhrman, B. et al., Ginger extract consumption reduces plasma cholesterol levels, inhibits LDL oxidation and attenuates development of atherosclerosis in the atherosclerotic apolipoprotein E deficient mice, *J. Nutr.,* 130, 1124, 2000.
17. Langley, P., Why a pomegranate? *BMJ,* 321, 1153, 2000.
18. Aviram, M., Polyphenols from pomegranate juice, red wine and licorice root protect against lipids peroxidation and attenuate cardiovascular diseases, in *Polyphenols 2000. 20th International Conference on Polyphenols*, Martens, S., Treutter, D., and Forkmann, G. (eds.), Freising-Weihenstephan, Germany, 158, 2002.

19. Gil, M.I. et al., Antioxidant activity of pomegranate juice and its relationship with phenolic composition and processing, *J. Agric. Food Chem.*, 48, 4581, 2000.
20. Ben Nasr, C., Ayed, N., and Metche, M., Quantitative determination of the polyphenolic content of pomegranate peel, *Z. Lebensm. Unters. Forsch.*, 203, 374, 1996.
21. Aviram, M., Pomegranate juice as a major source for polyphenolic flavonoids and it is most potent antioxidant against LDL oxidation and atherosclerosis, in *Proceedings of the 11th Biennial Meeting of the Society for Free Radical Research International* (Paris, July 16–20, 2002), by Monduzzi Editore S.p.A.—MEDIMOND, Inc., 523, 2002.
22. Aviram, M. et al., Pomegranate juice polyphenols decrease oxidative stress, low-density lipoprotein atherogenic modifications and atherosclerosis, *Free Radic. Res.*, 36 (Supplement 1), 72, 2002.
23. Aviram, M. et al., Pomegranate juice flavonoids inhibit low-density lipoprotein oxidation and cardiovascular diseases: Studies in atherosclerotic mice and in humans, *Drugs Ex. Clin. Res.*, 28, 49, 2002.
24. Cerda, B. et al., Evaluation of the bioavailability and metabolism in the rat of punicalagin, an antioxidant polyphenol from pomegranate juice, *Eur. J. Nutr.*, 42, 18, 2003.
25. Cerda, B. et al., Repeated oral administration of high doses of the pomegranate ellagitannin punicalagin to rats for 37 days is not toxic, *J. Agric. Food Chem.*, 51, 3493, 2003.
26. Seeram, N.P., Lee, R., and Heber, D., Bioavailability of ellagic acid in human plasma after consumption of ellagitannins from pomegranate (*Punica granatum* L.) juice, *Clin. Chim. Acta*, 348, 63, 2004.
27. Perez-Vicente, A., Gil-Izquierdo, A., and Garcia-Viguera, C., In vitro gastrointestinal digestion study of pomegranate juice phenolic compounds, anthocyanins, and vitamin C, *J. Agric. Food Chem.*, 50, 2308, 2002.
28. Aviram, M. et al., Pomegranate juice consumption reduces oxidative stress, atherogenic modifications to LDL, and platelet aggregation: Studies in humans and in the atherosclerotic apolipoprotein E-deficient mice, *Am. J. Clin. Nutr.*, 71, 1062, 2000.
29. Kaplan, M. et al., Pomegranate juice supplementation to atherosclerotic mice reduces macrophages lipid peroxidation, cellular cholesterol accumulation and development of atherosclerosis, *J. Nutr.*, 131, 2082, 2001.
30. de Nigris, F. et al., Beneficial effects of pomegranate juice on oxidation-sensitive genes and endothelial nitric oxide synthase activity at sites of perturbed shear stress, *Proc. Natl. Acad. Sci. USA*, 102, 4896, 2005.
31. Aviram, M. et al., Pomegranate juice consumption for 3 years by patients with carotid artery stenosis reduces common carotid intima-media thickness, blood pressure and LDL oxidation, *Clin. Nutr.*, 23, 423, 2004.
32. Rosenblat, M., Hayek, T., and Aviram, M., Antioxidative effects of pomegranate juice (PJ) consumption by diabetic patients on serum and on macrophages, *Atherosclerosis*, 187, 363, 2006.
33. Chidambara Murthy, K.N., Jayaprakasha, G.K., and Singh, R.P., Studies on antioxidant activity of pomegranate (*Punica granatum*) peel extract using in vivo models, *J. Agric. Food Chem.*, 50, 4791, 2002.
34. Aviram, M. et al., Human serum paraoxonase (PON1) is inactivated by oxidized low density lipoprotein and preserved by antioxidants, *Free Radic. Biol. Med.*, 26, 892, 1999.
35. Aviram, M., Review of human studies on oxidative damage and antioxidant protection related to cardiovascular diseases, *Free Radic. Res.*, 33, S85, 2000.
36. Berliner, J.A. et al., Atherosclerosis: Basic mechanisms: Oxidation, inflammation and genetics, *Circulation*, 9, 2488, 1995.

37. Fuhrman, B., Oiknine, J., and Aviram, M., Iron induces lipid peroxidation in cultured macrophages, increases their ability to oxidatively modify LDL and affect their secretory properties, *Atherosclerosis*, 111, 65, 1994.
38. Fuhrman, B. et al., Increased uptake of low density lipoprotein (LDL) by oxidized macrophages is the result of enhanced LDL receptor activity and of progressive LDL oxidation, *Free Radic. Biol. Med.*, 23, 34, 1997.
39. Fuhrman, B., Volkova, N., and Aviram, M., Oxidative stress increases the expression of the CD36 scavenger receptor and the cellular uptake of oxidized low-density lipoprotein in macrophages from atherosclerotic mice: Protective role of antioxidants and of paraoxonase, *Atherosclerosis*, 161, 307, 2002.
40. Aggarwal, B.B., and Shishoda, S., Suppression of the nuclear factor-{kappa}B activation pathway by spice-derived phytochemicals: Reasoning for seasoning, *Ann. NY Acad. Sci.*, 1030, 434, 2004.
41. Schubert, S.Y., Neeman, I., and Resnick, N., A novel mechanism for the inhibition of NF-kappaB activation in vascular endothelial cells by natural antioxidants, *FASEB J.*, 16, 1931, 2002.
42. Schubert, S.Y., Lansky, E.P., and Neeman, I., Antioxidant and eicosanoid enzyme inhibition properties of pomegranate seed oil and fermented juice flavonoids, *J. Ethnopharmacol.*, 66, 11, 1999.
43. Aviram, M., Interaction of oxidized low density lipoprotein with macrophages in atherosclerosis and the anti-atherogenicity of antioxidants, *Eur. J. Clin. Chem. Clin. Biochem.*, 34, 599, 1996.
44. Steinberg, D., Low density lipoprotein oxidation and its pathobiological significance, *J. Biol. Chem.*, 272, 20963, 1997.
45. Goldstein, J.L., and Brown, M.S., Regulation of the mevalonate pathway, *Nature*, 343, 425, 1990.
46. Brown, M.S., and Goldstein, J.L., A receptor-mediated pathway for cholesterol homeostasis, *Science*, 232, 34, 1986.
47. Krieger, M., The best of cholesterols, the worst of cholesterols: A tale of two receptors, *Proc. Natl. Acad. Sci. USA*, 4, 4077, 1998.
48. Fuhrman, B., Volkova, N., and Aviram, M., Pomegranate juice inhibits oxidized LDL uptake and cholesterol biosynthesis in macrophages, *J. Nutr. Biochem.*, 16, 570, 2005.
49. Rozenberg, O., Howell, A., and Aviram, M., Pomegranate juice sugar fraction reduces macrophage oxidative state, whereas white grape juice sugar fraction increases it, *Atherosclerosis*, 188, 68, 2006.
50. Shiner, M., Fuhrman, B., and Aviram, M., Macrophage paraoxonase 2 (PON2) expression is up-regulated by pomegranate juice phenolic antioxidants via PPAR gamma and AP-1 pathway activation, *Atherosclerosis*, 198, 313, 2006.
51. Seeram N. et al., Rapid large scale purification of ellagitannins from pomegranate husk, a by-product of the commercial juice industry, *Separation Purification Technol.*, 41, 49, 2005.
52. Rosenblat M., Volkova N., Coleman R., and Aviram M., Pomegranate by-product administration to apolipoprotein E-deficient mice attenuates atherosclerosis development as a result of decreased macrophage oxidative stress and reduced cellular uptake of oxidized low-density lipoprotein, *J. Agric. Food. Chem.*, 54, 1928, 2006.

CHAPTER 9

Customizing Dietary Recommendations by Genotype in the Era of Genomics

Sina Vakili, Grace Jooyoung Shin, and Marie A. Caudill

CONTENTS

INTRODUCTION

The completion of the Human Genome Project marked the beginning of the "genomic era." The complete DNA sequence of the "average" human is now known along with specific nuances in the genetic code that may influence disease risk, responses to pharmacological agents, and nutrient tolerances and requirements. Single nucleotide polymorphisms (SNPs), changes in a single base pair that exist in more than 1% of the population, are the most prevalent form of genetic variability in the human genome. SNPs occur about every 1000 base pairs representing about three million differences between individuals' DNA. Of interest to scientists are the small fraction (~240,000–400,000 common variants) that may be responsible for the genetic component of differences in health, behavior, and other human traits.[1]

Although the human genome project and subsequent efforts have sparked interest in the effects of SNPs on common diseases, the intersection of genomics and nutrition is relatively unexplored. To this end, nutritional genomics has emerged as a discipline that seeks to provide information on gene–nutrient interactions (and vice versa) that may allow for customization of a diet based on a particular genotype. Nutritional genomics encompasses nutrigenetics, the influence of genetic variation on nutrient tolerances and requirements, and nutrigenomics (the influence of nutrients on the human genome).

The objective of this chapter is to examine the feasibility, within the context of our current state of inquiry into gene–nutrient interactions, of using genetic information as cues upon which to base specific nutritional recommendations. This chapter is an extension of our previous communication entitled "Personalized Nutrition: Nutritional Genomics as a Potential Tool for Targeted Medical Nutrition Therapy."[2] Our approach is to explore the influence of common genetic variants within heart susceptibility genes on cardiovascular disease risk and to assess the role, if any, of using these variants as genetic cues for making specific dietary recommendations.

CANDIDATE GENES FOR CORONARY ARTERY DISEASE

Coronary artery disease (CAD) is the most common form of cardiovascular disease, is multifactorial and polygenic, and is usually caused by atherosclerosis. CAD is characterized by a narrowing of the coronary arteries that prevents an adequate supply of blood to the heart muscle and is associated with inflammation,[3,4] dyslipidemia,[5] and/or hyperhomocysteinemia.[6] Thus, genes that have the potential to modulate such factors (i.e., inflammation) represent viable choices for heart health susceptibility genes. In our previous report, we included an analysis of genes involved in homocysteine metabolism (i.e., methylenetetrahydrofolate reductase), lipid metabolism (i.e., cholesteryl ester transfer protein, lipoprotein lipase, apolipoprotein C-III), and inflammation (interleukin 6). We now report on apolipoproteins (apo) A-I and A-IV and tumor necrosis factor alpha (TNF-α), genes involved in lipid metabolism and inflammation, respectively.[2] A summary of the key findings presented in this chapter, including the influence of relevant genetic variants on CAD risk and possible customized dietary recommendations for those carrying the variant allele, is depicted in Table 9.1.

Apolipoprotein (Apo) A-I

Apolipoprotein A-I is the main protein found in high-density lipoprotein (HDL) and is synthesized mainly in the liver and small intestine[7,8] as a single 243 amino acid polypeptide chain.[9] Apo A-I is a key component of the reverse cholesterol transport process[10] and is an activator of lecithin cholesterol acyltransferase.[11] HDL and apo A-I may also have antioxidant, antithrombotic, and anti-inflammatory properties, which could have important anti-atherogenic effects.[12] In humans there seems to be an inverse relationship between apo A-I levels and risk of CAD,[13–15] suggesting that apo A-I is cardioprotective. Thus, functional polymorphisms in the apo A-I gene that affect gene expression or protein activity are of interest.

A region on the long arm of chromosome 11q23-q24 encodes for the apo A-I gene along with apo C-III and apo A-IV genes.[16] The 3′ end of the apo A-I gene lies

Table 9.1 Summary of Discussed Single Nucleotide Polymorphisms, Including Their Influence on the Risk of Coronary Artery Disease and Some Possible Medical Nutrition Therapy Recommendations

Gene	SNP	Allele Frequency[a]	Influence of Variant	Effect on CAD Risk	Possible MNT Recommendation
Apo A-I	-75G→A	14–22%[19,20]	↑ apo A-I/↑ HDL [22,24–26,30] No/opposite effect[23,27–29,31–33]	↑ Risk[29,31,32] No effect[33]	↑ PUFA (women)[34] Low-fat diets (men)[19]
Apo A-IV	360G→T	5–12%[47,48]	↓ TG[60,56]/↓ LDL[61]/↑ HDL[47] No/opposite effect[52,53,62–65]	No effect[44,68]	↑ Unsaturated fats[76,77] Avoidance of low-fat diets[76]
Apo A-IV	347A→T	22%[55,56]	↓ LDL[52,63]/↓ TG (females)[70] ↑ LDL[61]/↑ TG (males)[70] No effect[66,60,64,65,7,72] Possible ↓ of antioxidant status[44]	↑ Risk[b,44]	↑ Unsaturated fats[78,79]
TNFα	-308G→A	17%[94]	↑ TNFα[90,91] No TNFα effect[92] ↑ CRP[93]	↑ Risk[c,97–99] No effect[95,96]	↑ Fish oil[92] ↑ Soy[100] ↑ Caffeine[101]

a Approximate frequency in Caucasian populations.
b Possibly through a mechanism unrelated to lipid transport.
c Influenced by obesity/diabetes and/or presence of C4A*Q0 allele.

2.6 and 10 kb from the apo CIII and apo AIV genes, respectively.[16] Among numerous genetic variants within the apo A-I gene, the -75G→A promoter genetic variant is the most widely studied. This polymorphic marker abolishes an MspI restriction site and is commonly referred to as the M1 variant. The prevalence of the -75G→A SNP differs among ethnic and racial groups with a frequency of 30% in East Asian populations, such as Taiwanese, Chinese, and Malaysian,[17,18] compared to approximately 14–22% in Caucasian populations [19,20] and ~10% in Nigerian populations.[21] The variant A allele is associated with increased transcription efficiency in some studies[22] and decreased efficiency in others.[23]

The influence of the G→A substitution at -75 of the apo A-I gene on biomarkers (i.e., apo A-I and HDL-cholesterol) of CAD risk is inconclusive. There is a similar number of studies reporting a significant elevating effect of the A allele (relative to the GG genotype) on HDL and/or apo A-I[24–26]as those reporting no association.[27–29] In a meta-analysis including 3060 healthy individuals, the polymorphism was associated with a minor but significant elevating effect on apo A-I levels,[30] suggesting that the A allele may confer some protection against CAD.

However, among the relatively few studies that have assessed the influence of the -75 A allele on CAD outcome, most have reported a deleterious influence. Reguero et al. reported a higher frequency of the -75A allele in male patients from Spain with a diagnosis of CAD and fewer than 50 years of age.[31] Wang et al. reported more severe CAD in an Australian coronary population for patients homozygous for the variant -75A allele.[29] Similarly, Chabra et al. reported that carriers of the A allele were approximately four times as likely to develop triple vessel disease compared to individuals with the GG genotype.[32] However, Ordovas et al. reported no difference in the prevalence of the A allele among CAD cases and controls of the U.S. Framingham cohort.[33] In all of these studies assessing the relationship between the G→A polymorphism on CAD, HDL-cholesterol did not differ significantly between the -75G→A genotypes [29,31,33] or was lower in carriers of the A allele relative to the GG genotype.[32]

Several factors are likely contributors to the inconsistent findings related to the -75G→A polymorphism and CAD risk. Among these factors are gender and ethnicity differences, sample size bias when small sample sizes are used, presence of this polymorphism in different haplotypes, and environmental interactions. In regard to gene–environment interactions, Sigurdsson et al. reported that the -75A allele was only associated with increased HDL-cholesterol or apo A-I concentrations in non-smoking men.[26]

Gene–nutrient interactions have also been reported and appear to explain in part the highly variable data regarding the influence of this SNP on lipoproteins and CAD. Ordovos et al. examined whether fat intake modified the association between the -75A variant and HDL-cholesterol and/or apo A-I concentrations in 755 men and 822 women from the Framingham Offspring Study.[34] In women, a significant interaction was observed between the G-75A genotype and polyunsaturated fatty acids. When polyunsaturated fatty acid intake was <4% of energy, GG subjects had ~14% higher HDL-cholesterol than did carriers of the A allele. However, when polyunsaturated fatty acid intake was >8%, carriers of the A allele had ~13% higher

HDL-cholesterol than did the GG genotype. In men, the relationship was more complex with the polyunsaturated fatty acid intake effect only significant when interactions with alcohol consumption and tobacco smoking were also considered. In another study, men (36 GG, 14 GA) were fed a low-fat diet for 25 days, followed by a diet high in monounsaturated fatty acids for 28 days.[35] No differences in the lipoproteins were observed between the genotypes at baseline or at any other study time. However, a significant diet by genotype interaction was observed after consumption of the diet rich in monounsaturated fatty acids. Plasma low-density lipoprotein (LDL)-cholesterol increased significantly in subjects with the GA genotype but not in subjects with the GG genotype. Other data show that despite differences in lipoproteins between GG and GA genotypes, both respond favorably to a low-fat diet.[19] Overall, these data suggest that the rare A allele interacts with fat intake to influence lipoproteins.

Interesting research assessing the influence of select nutrients on apo A-I expression has been published (reviewed in Mooradian et al.[36]). Among some of the nutrients associated with decreased expression of the apo A-I gene in cell culture or animal models are polyunsaturated fatty acids, trans-fatty acids, omega-3 fatty acids, glucose, antioxidant vitamins, and zinc deficiency. In contrast, monounsaturated fatty acids, soy proteins, alcohol, and copper deficiency are associated with increased expression of the human apo A-I gene.

In summary, apolipoprotein A-I is important in reverse cholesterol transport and is needed for the proper assembly of HDL. The -75G→A polymorphism of the apo A-I gene is the most widely studied genetic variant in the apo A-I gene; however, data are inconclusive regarding the influence of this SNP on CAD risk. Among several factors that may contribute to the inconsistencies among studies are gene–environment and gene–nutrient interactions. Although it is clear that more studies are needed, existing data suggest that women carrying the A allele may benefit from a diet high in polyunsaturated fatty acid, while men carrying the A allele may benefit from a low-fat diet.

Apolipoprotein A-IV

Apo A-IV is a 46-kDa intestinal protein that is synthesized during lipid absorption and incorporated into the surface of nascent chylomicrons, which are subsequently secreted into lymph. In the lymphatic system, the majority of apo A-IV is displaced by apolipoprotein E and C-II (reviewed in Weinberg[37]), after which ~70% associates with HDL-cholesterol.[38] Apo C-II activates lipoprotein lipase (LPL) and is essential to hydrolysis of chylomicrons. Following lipolysis, chylomicron remnants are cleared from circulation by the apo E receptor. The apo A-IV protein appears to be important in chylomicron synthesis, triglyceride-rich lipoprotein metabolism, and the reverse cholesterol process. Data from *in vitro* studies suggest that apo A-IV is an important activator of lecithin cholesterol acyltransferase (LCAT)[39,40] and cholesteryl ester transfer protein (CETP).[41] Apo A-IV also influences triglyceride metabolism by mediating the transfer of apo C-II from HDL to chylomicrons, enhancing the activation of LPL.[42] In humans there seems to be an inverse relationship between apo A-IV levels and risk of CAD,[43–45] suggesting that apo A-IV is anti-atherogenic. Polymorphisms of the apo A-IV gene are of interest because of its involvement in both triglyceride and cholesterol metabolism.

The apo A-IV gene is located on the long arm of chromosome 11 near to apo C-III and apo A-I. Most published work on apo A-IV polymorphisms has focused on a G→T exchange at nucleotide position 2387 (third base of codon 360), which causes a glutamine to histidine substitution in the protein product.[46] The normal and variant apo A-IV proteins were originally detected by isoelectric focusing and are often referred to as apo A-IV-1 and apo A-IV-2 isoforms/alleles, respectively.[47] The prevalence of the G→T variant at codon 360 is ~5–12% in white populations.[47,48] Its sporadic distribution throughout nonwhite populations is thought to be through white admixture.[49] Nonwhite populations such as Nigerian blacks (0–3%), Japanese (0.1%), and Asian Indians (3%) have significantly lower frequencies.[50–53]

Another widely studied apo A-IV SNP is an A→T polymorphism at nucleotide 2346 (first base of codon 347), which causes a threonine-to-serine substitution in the protein product.[54,55] The A→T variant at codon 347 occurs at almost double the frequency of the 360G→T variant with a prevalence of ~22% in Caucasian populations.[55,56] However, ethnic differences have been described with lower frequencies in African blacks (9.5%) and Hispanic populations (12.9%).[53] The 360G→T and 347A→T genetic variants are in strong linkage disequilibrium and tend not to occur together.[55,57]

It is of interest to note that the 360T variant increases the lipid affinity of the protein product, which in turn inhibits the exchange of apo E and apo C-II and delays postprandial intravascular clearance of triglyceride-rich lipoproteins.[58] In contrast, the 347T variant allele facilitates postprandial intravascular clearance of triglyceride-rich lipoproteins[59] and is predicted to decrease the lipid affinity of the protein product and enhance the exchange of apo E and apo C-II. Thus, the antagonistic interaction between these two SNPs may affect the magnitude of postprandial triglyceride response[37] in persons with combined heterozygosity for both variants (i.e., 360 GT and 347 AT). In turn, if the polymorphisms are linked to CAD risk through an effect on lipid metabolism, the influence of either polymorphism is likely to be strongly dependent upon the presence of the other.

For the apo A-IV codon 360G→T polymorphism, some studies have shown a more favorable lipid profile, such as decreased triglycerides[60] and LDL-cholesterol,[61] as well as increased HDL-cholesterol.[47] However, others have failed to observe these associations or have shown opposite effects.[52,53,62–66] To further explore the relationship between the 360G→T variant and biomarkers of CAD, Cendorogolo and others combined their data from the Framingham Offspring Study with several others and performed a meta-analysis.[66] After exclusion of studies that included subjects with CAD or diabetes mellitus, the codon 360T variant was associated with a significantly lower level of triglycerides (–13.1 mg/dL). The triglyceride-lowering effect may suggest that the T allele is associated with greater activation of LCAT and/or LPL than the G allele.[67]

Few studies have examined the influence of the G→T polymorphism in codon 360 on CAD. In a prospectively designed study involving 2808 healthy middle-aged men from the United Kingdom, the codon 360G→T polymorphism was found not to influence CAD risk.[44] Another study reported that the apo A-IV codon 360G→T was not a determinant of predisposition to CAD in a European study population consisting of 1261 controls and 629 cases, defined as students whose fathers had myocardial infarction before 55 years of age.[68] However, in populations more prone to hyperlipidemia (i.e., diabetes and obesity),[69] the 360T allele could be pro-atherogenic due to its role in delaying clearance of postprandial triglyceride-rich lipoproteins.[37]

Like the 360T allele, results for the biochemical effect of the 347A→T variant have been inconsistent. Some studies have shown decreases in LDL-cholesterol,[52,63] while another showed an increase.[61] Herron et al. reported lower triglycerides in female carriers of the variant 347T allele and higher triglycerides in male carriers of the variant 347T allele relative to noncarriers.[70] However, most studies have shown no effect on lipid or lipoprotein levels.[56,60,64,65,71,72] There has been speculation, though, that the influence of the apo A-IV 347A→T on CAD may be independent of its effect on lipids. In a prospective study of 2808 healthy middle-aged men from the United Kingdom, homozygotes for the 347T allele were twice as likely to experience a clinically defined CAD event compared to men homozygous for the wild-type 347A allele.[44] The risk was independent of any lipid parameter, suggesting a mechanism unrelated to reverse cholesterol transport.[44] In this same study, Wong et al. examined the relationship between the 347T variant and plasma apo A-IV concentrations in 1600 healthy young European men and women and observed significantly lower apo A-IV levels in homozygotes for the variant 347T allele compared with carriers of the 347A allele.[44] Given the potential antioxidant properties of the apo A-IV protein,[73] it was suggested that individuals homozygous for the 347T allele may have reduced antioxidant status, increased oxidative stress, and increased CAD risk relative to 347A allele carriers.[44]

Dietary intervention studies suggest that the 360T variant allele delays postprandial plasma triglyceride clearance.[58] Postprandial triglyceride concentrations in carriers of the 360T variant allele were significantly higher between 2 and 5 hours in plasma, chylomicrons, and VLDL and peaked at 3 hours versus 2 hours for the GG subjects.[58] The 360T allele is also associated with decreased mean fractional cholesterol absorption in subjects with the 347AA genotype and consuming a high polyunsaturated fat diet.[74] Nonetheless, these alterations in lipid absorption and metabolism do not always translate to changes in lipoprotein patterns. Initial work suggested that the 360T variant attenuated the response of LDL-cholesterol to increased dietary cholesterol intake. McCombs et al. reported a smaller increase in LDL-cholesterol among 11 (eight men, three women) 360 G→T carriers versus 12 (nine men, three women) noncarriers (19 mg/dL vs. 1 mg/dL; $p = 0.03$) when subjects increased their cholesterol intake from about 200 to about 1100 mg/day by the addition of four egg yolks per day.[75] However, subsequent work suggested that the effects of the variant allele on LDL-cholesterol response to changes in cholesterol intake may be weak relative to the effect of the fatty acid. In this regard, Weinberg et al. reported that the apo A-IV genotype did not influence LDL-cholesterol response to fat-modified diets, despite an almost threefold increase in cholesterol.[74] Thus, when there is a change in dietary saturated fatty acid or polyunsaturated fatty acids, the fatty acid effects on LDL-cholesterol may predominate and partially (or totally) abolish the effect of the allele.[37]

The 360T variant allele may influence HDL-cholesterol response to changes in cholesterol and/or fat. Jansen et al. reported that HDL-cholesterol decreased by 1 mg/dL in 33 GG individuals and by 10 mg/dL in eight GT individuals after switching from a high saturated fat diet to a low-fat diet.[76] However, on the high monounsaturated fat diet, HDL-cholesterol increased by 1 mg/dL in the GG individuals and by 10 mg/dL in the GT individuals ($p = 0.003$). Wallace et al. reported that HDL-cholesterol increased in the six subjects with the GT genotype when polyunsaturated fatty acids replaced saturated fatty acids, whereas it decreased in the 30 subjects with GG genotype ($p = 0.03$).[77] Taken together, these data suggest that carriers of the 360T allele may benefit from a diet rich in unsaturated fats, whereas a low-fat diet may be contraindicated for these individuals in regard to HDL-cholesterol.

Considering the anti-atherosclerotic roles of apo A-IV, any dietary intervention that may increase apo A-IV levels would be of interest. Some of the most encouraging studies have found that isolated fatty acids can regulate expression and production of apo A-IV in enterocytes.[78,79] In a human cell culture model, Stan et al. demonstrated that docosahexaenoic and oleic acids were potent activators of apo A-IV gene expression and synthesis.[78] The mRNA levels of apo A-IV were about 140 and 160% higher than controls for docosahexaenoic and oleic acids, respectively, after a 20-hour incubation period. In a human study involving 48 healthy men and women, Kratz et al. reported that consumption of diets rich in unsaturated fats (olive oil, canola oil, or sunflower oil) increased plasma apo A-IV levels by about 16%, regardless of apo A-IV genotype or gender.[79] It remains to be established, however, if dietary stimulation of apo A-IV lowers the risk of CAD.

In summary, apo A-IV, like its close neighbors apo A-I and C-III, is an important protein of the lipid transport system. Levels of apo A-IV are inversely correlated with CAD risk and numerous studies have investigated the influence of genetic polymorphisms within this gene on lipid and lipoprotein levels. The biochemical consequences of having the G→T substitution at codon 360 are controversial, but there is limited evidence that having this variant in a cardiosensitive state (i.e., diabetes) may increase the risk of CAD. The influence of the A→T substitution at codon 347 on lipoprotein patterns is also controversial, but existing data suggest that variant 347T allele may be increasing CAD risk through a mechanism that is unrelated to lipid transport. Dietary intervention studies have shown that LDL-cholesterol levels are less responsive to changes in dietary cholesterol among carriers of the 360T allele. However, the allele effect may be abolished when fatty acid intake is also manipulated. In regard to HDL-cholesterol, data suggest that carriers of the variant 360T allele may benefit from a diet rich in unsaturated fat, whereas a low-fat diet may be contraindicated. Initial findings of nutrigenomic studies reveal that apo A-IV gene expression may be increased with certain fatty acids. Such findings may be useful in medical nutrition therapy if future investigations demonstrate that increasing apo A-IV decreases CAD.

Tumor Necrosis Factor Alpha (TNF-α)

TNF-α is a multifunctional pro-inflammatory cytokine that is synthesized as a membrane protein and subsequently cleaved to a soluble 17-kDa form.[80] Systemic or local inflammation triggers the production of TNF-α mostly by macrophages but also by adipocytes, monocytes, and muscle tissue.[81] Production of TNF-α, in turn, stimulates the production of interleukin 6, which induces hepatic production of acute phase reactants, including C-reactive protein (CRP).[82] A meta-analysis of seven prospective studies (1053 cases) reported that the risk ratio for CAD was 1.7 for people with CRP levels in the highest tertile compared to those in the lowest.[83] In addition to having a critical role in CAD risk prediction, emerging data support a possible causatory role of CRP in the development and progression of CAD (reviewed in Wilson et al.[84]). Elevated levels of TNF-α have also been linked to CAD. In a cohort of 81-year-old humans, high levels of TNF-α in the blood were associated with a high prevalence of atherosclerosis.[85] In addition, serum TNF-α levels are associated with carotid atherosclerosis in healthy men[86] and an increased risk of recurrent coronary events in survivors of myocardial infarction.[87] Moreover, TNF-α mRNA has been found in hearts of ischemic heart disease and end-stage dilated cardiomyopathy as well as atherosclerotic plaques,[88,89] suggesting a direct contribution to the atherosclerotic process. Because TNF-α has a central role in the inflammatory process, genetic polymorphisms that alter the expression and level of TNF-α represent strong candidates as CAD susceptibility alleles.

The TNF-α gene is located on chromosome 6 at p21 between the class I and III clusters of the human major histocompatibility complex.[80] The TNF-α gene is highly polymorphic, especially in the 5' region.[80] The most widely studied genetic variant in the TNF-α gene is the -308G→A genetic variant located in the promoter region. *In vitro* studies have shown that the variant -308A allele is associated with increased transcription of the TNF-α gene resulting in higher protein levels,[90,91] although this has not been found in all studies.[92] The -308A allele is also associated with elevated plasma CRP concentrations.[93] In a study involving 456 white (225 men, 231 women) and 232 black (83 men, 149 women) healthy adults, AA homozygotes for the -308G→A variant had higher baseline CRP levels than other genotypes in white men ($p = 0.001$), black men ($p = 0.044$), and black women ($p = 0.032$).[93] The lack of association in white women was largely explained by fatness. Heterozygosity for the variant occurs in 16.7% of the population, whereas the homozygosity for the AA genotype is generally below 2.5%.[94]

Although numerous studies have investigated the influence of the TNF-α -308G→A polymorphism on autoimmune diseases (reviewed in Hajeer and Hutchinson[80]), fewer have investigated its influence on CAD risk. In a European population, Herrmann et al. investigated patients with CAD ($n = 641$) and found no association between the TNF-α -308A allele and susceptibility to the disease relative to the controls ($n = 710$).[95] However, the TNF-α -308A was associated with parental history of myocardial infarction. In an autopsy series study conducted in 700 Caucasian Finnish men aged 33–70 years, Keso et al. found no association between TNF-α -308 polymorphism and CAD, although it was noted that more extensive morphometric atherosclerotic changes seemed to be associated with the rare -308 AA genotype.[96] Padovani et al. reported that the TNF-α -308A allele may increase the risk of myocardial infarction conferred by obesity in a Brazilian population.[97] In this regard, the odds ratio for myocardial infarction for obese carriers of the A allele (13 patients, one control) was 14.5 versus 2.8 for obese noncarriers (28 patients, 11 controls), although this was not significant, probably due to the small subject number.[97] Vendrell et al. reported that in a Mediterranean population with type 2 diabetes, the A allele was significantly associated with the presence of CAD, particularly among women.[98] The odds ratio for CAD among type 2 diabetic patients in the presence of the -308A allele was 2.9 and increased to 4.3 if only women were considered.

Taken together, these data suggest that the influence of the variant allele may be dependent on the existence of other diseases. Data also suggest that the influence of the -308A allele on CAD may be dependent upon the presence of the nonexpressed variants of the C4 genes, components of the classical complement pathway. Szalai et al. reported that the risk of having CAD was 3.2 times higher in patients with TNF-α -308A + C4A*Q0 alleles than with TNF-α -308A without C4A*Q0. Moreover, the risk of having CAD was 2.5 times higher in patients with TNF-α -308A + C4A*Q0 alleles than with TNF-α -308G + C4A*Q0 allelic combination.[99]

Few studies have assessed the influence of the TNF-α -308G→A variant on the response to dietary components. However, one study reported that among healthy men with the highest levels of presupplementation (i.e., baseline) TNF-α production in peripheral blood mononuclear cells, carriers of the -308A allele experienced significantly greater declines in TNF-α production after fish oil supplementation (6 g/d for 12 weeks) than noncarriers.[92] Paradoxically, however, among men with the lowest levels of presupplementation TNF-α production, production increased significantly after fish oil supplementation, regardless of TNF-α -308G→A genotype.

In addition to fish oil, nutrigenomic studies have identified other possible modulators of TNF-α production and/or release in vitro. Kang et al. reported that soybean saponins suppressed the release of TNF-α by LPS-stimulated murine peritoneal macrophages.[100] Horrigan et al. demonstrated that concentrations of caffeine that were relevant to human consumption consistently suppressed the production of TNF-α in human blood.[101] Clearly, more studies that address the anti-inflammatory effects of food components in studies involving humans are warranted.

In summary, TNF-α is an inflammatory cytokine that induces the production of C-reactive protein. Elevated levels of TNF-α and C-reactive protein in plasma are associated with increased risk of CAD. The TNF-α -308 G→A polymorphism is generally associated with greater expression of the TNF-α gene and higher levels of C-reactive protein. Data are equivocal on the relationship between the -308G→A genetic variant and CAD risk. However, in the presence of other diseases, such as diabetes and obesity, the -308A allele appears to increase risk. Given the possible increased production of TNF-α, people who carry the -308A allele may benefit from increased consumption of food components shown to exert anti-inflammatory effects in humans.

CONCLUDING COMMENTS

Although it is relatively easy to find single studies that demonstrate an effect of a variant allele on disease outcome and/or an interaction between a variant allele and a dietary component, it is rare to find consistency among studies. Most studies assessing the influence of genetic variation on disease risk and/or nutrient requirements/ tolerances have taken a genotype rather than haplotype approach. In this regard, the SNP under investigation may belong to a haplotype with protective effects as well as to a different haplotype with detrimental effects. The complexity of gene–nutrient interactions also underscores the difficulty in replicating and interpreting study findings. The influence of a genetic variant on the response of a given biomarker to a dietary treatment is affected not only by what is included in the diet but also by what is excluded (i.e., foods high in cholesterol, saturated fatty acids, etc.). Thus, one of the greatest challenges of using genetic information as cues for targeted medical nutrition therapy will be determining when enough is known to act in a preemptive manner.

ACKNOWLEDGMENTS

This chapter was supported by NIH grant no. S06GM53933 and funds from the California Agricultural Research Initiative.

REFERENCES

1. Cargill M, Altshuler D, Ireland J et al. Characterization of single-nucleotide polymorphisms in coding regions of human genes. *Nat Gen.* 1999, 22:231–238.
2. Vakili S, Caudill MA. Personalized nutrition: Nutritional genomics as a potential tool for targeted medical nutrition therapy. *Nutr Rev.* 2007, 65:301–315.
3. Ross R. Atherosclerosis—An inflammatory disease. *N Engl J Med.* 1999, 340:115–126.
4. Steffens S, Mach F. Inflammation and atherosclerosis. *Herz.* 2004, 29:741–748.
5. LaRosa JC, Hnninghake Du, Bush D, Grundy et al. The cholesterol facts. A summary of the evidence relating dietary fats, serum cholesterol, and coronary heart disease. A joint statement by the American Heart Association and the National Heart, Lung, and Blood Institute. The Task Force on Cholesterol Issues, American Heart Association. *Circulation.* 1990, 8:1721–1733.
6. The Homocysteine Studies Collaboration. Homocysteine and risk of ischemic heart disease and stroke: A meta-analysis. *JAMA.* 2002, 288:2015–2022.
7. Schonfeld G, Bell E, Alpers DH. Intestinal apoproteins during fat absorption. *J Clin Invest.* 1978, 61:1539–1550.
8. Zannis VI, Breslow JL, SanGiacomo TR, Aden DP, Knowles BB. Characterization of the major apolipoproteins secreted by two human hepatoma cell lines. *Biochemistry.* 1981, 20:7089–7096.

9. Karathanasis SK, Zannis VI, Breslow JL. Isolation and characterization of the human apolipoprotein A-I gene. *Proc Natl Acad Sci USA.* 1983, 80:6147–6151.
10. Reichl D, Miller NE. Pathophysiology of reverse cholesterol transport. Insights from inherited disorders of lipoprotein metabolism. *Arteriosclerosis.* 1989, 9:785–797.
11. Fielding CJ, Shore VG, Fielding PE. A protein cofactor of lecithin: Cholesteryl acyl-transferase. *Biochem Biophys Res Commun.* 1972, 46:1493–1498.
12. Mooradian AD, Haas MJ, Wadud K. Ascorbic acid and alpha-tocopherol down-regulate apolipoprotein A-I gene expression in HepG2 and Caco-2 cell lines. *Metabolism.* 2006, 55:159–167.
13. Maciejko JJ, Holmes DR, Kottke BA, Zinsmeister AR, Dinh DM, Mao SJ. Apolipoprotein A-I as a marker of angiographically assessed coronary-artery disease. *N Engl J Med.* 1983, 309:385–389.
14. Forte TM, McCall MR. The role of apolipoprotein A-I-containing lipoproteins in atherosclerosis. *Curr Opin Lipidiol.* 1994, 5:354–364.
15. Stampfer MJ, Sacks FM, Salvini S, Willett WC, Hennekens CH. A prospective study of cholesterol, apolipoproteins, and the risk of myocardial infarction. *N Engl J Med.* 1991, 325: 373–381.
16. Karathanasis SK. Apolipoprotein multigene family. Tandem organization of human apolipoprotein AI, CIII, and AIV genes. *Proc Natl Acad Sci USA.* 1985, 82:6374–6378.
17. Wu JH, Kao JT, Wen MS, Lo SK. DNA polymorphisms at the apolipoprotein A1-CIII loci in Taiwanese: Correlation of plasma APOCIII with triglyceride level and body mass index. *J Formos Med Assoc.* 2000, 99:367–374.
18. Heng, CK, Low, PS, Saha, N. Variations in the promoter region of the apolipoprotein A-I gene influence plasma lipoprotein(a) levels in Asian Indian neonates from Singapore. *Pediatr. Res.* 2001, 49:514–518.
19. Carmena-Ramon RF, Ordovas JM, Ascaso JF, Real J, Priego MA, Carmena R. Influence of genetic variation at the apo A-I gene locus on lipid levels and response to diet in familial hypercholesterolemia. *Atherosclerosis.* 1998, 139:107–113.
20. Wang XL, Badenhop R, Humphrey KE, Wilcken DE. New MspI polymorphism at +83 bp of the human apolipoprotein AI gene: Association with increased circulating high density lipoprotein cholesterol levels. *Genet Epidemiol.* 1996, 13:1–10.
21. Kamboh MI, Bunker CH, Aston CE et al. Genetic association of five apolipoprotein polymorphisms with serum lipoprotein-lipid levels in African blacks. *Genet Epidemiol.* 1999, 16:205–222.
22. Angotti E, Mele E, Costanzo F, Avvedimento EV. A polymorphism (G→A transition) in –78 position of apolipoprotein A-I promoter increases transcription efficiency. *J Biol Chem.* 1994, 269:17371–17374.
23. Smith JD, Brinton EA, Breslow JL. Polymorphism in the human apolipoprotein A-I gene promoter region. Association of the minor allele with decreased production rate *in vivo* and promoter activity *in vitro. J Clin Invest.* 1992, 89:1796–1800.
24. Jeenah M, Kessling A, Miller N, Humphries S. G to A substitution in the promoter region of the apolipoprotein AI gene is associated with elevated serum apolipoprotein AI and high density lipoprotein cholesterol concentrations. *Mol Biol Med.* 1990, 7:233–241.
25. Paul-Hayase H, Rosseneu M, Robinson D, Van Bervliet JP, Deslypere JP, Humphries SE. Polymorphisms in the apolipoprotein (apo) AI-CIII-AIV gene cluster: Detection of genetic variation determining plasma apo AI, apo CIII and apo AIV concentrations. *Hum Genet.* 1992, 88:439–446.

26. Sigurdsson G, Jr, Gudnason V, Sigurdsson G, Humphries SE. Interaction between a polymorphism of the apo A-I promoter region and smoking determines plasma levels of HDL and apo A-I. *Arterioscler Thromb.* 1992, 12:1017–1022.

27. Larson IA, Ordovas JM, Barnard JR et al. Effects of apolipoprotein A-I genetic variations on plasma apolipoprotein, serum lipoprotein and glucose levels. *Clin Genet.* 2002, 61:176–184.

28. Ma YQ, Thomas GN, Tomlinson B. Association of two apolipoprotein A-I gene MspI polymorphisms with lipid and blood pressure levels. *Int J Cardiol.* 2005, 102:309–314.

29. Wang XL, Liu SX, McCredie RM, Wilcken DE. Polymorphisms at the 5′-end of the apolipoprotein AI gene and severity of coronary artery disease. *J Clin Invest.* 1996, 98:372–377.

30. Juo SH, Wyszynski DF, Beaty TH, Huang HY, Bailey-Wilson JE. Mild association between the A/G polymorphism in the promoter of the apolipoprotein A-I gene and apolipoprotein A-I levels: A meta-analysis. *Am J Med Genet.* 1999, 82:235–241.

31. Reguero JR, Cubero GI, Batalla A et al. Apolipoprotein A1 gene polymorphisms and risk of early coronary disease. *Cardiology.* 1998, 90:231–235.

32. Chabra S, Narang R, Lakshmy R, Das N. APOA1-75 G to A substitution associated with severe forms of CAD, lower levels of HDL and apoA-I among Northern Indians. *Dis Markers.* 2005, 21:169–174.

33. Ordovas JM, Civeira F, Genest J, Jr et al. Restriction fragment length polymorphisms of the apolipoprotein A-I, C-III, A-IV gene locus. Relationships with lipids, apolipoproteins, and premature coronary artery disease. *Atherosclerosis.* 1991, 87:75–86.

34. Ordovas JM, Corella D, Cupples LA et al. Polyunsaturated fatty acids modulate the effects of the APOA1 G-A polymorphism on HDL-cholesterol concentrations in a sex-specific manner: The Framingham Study. *Am J Clin Nutr.* 2002, 75:38–46.

35. Lopez-Miranda J, Ordovas JM, Espino A et al. Influence of mutation in human apolipoprotein A-1 gene promoter on plasma LDL cholesterol response to dietary fat. *Lancet.* 1994, 343:1246–1249.

36. Mooradian AD, Haas MJ, Wong NC. The effect of select nutrients on serum high-density lipoprotein cholesterol and apolipoprotein A-I levels. *Endocr Rev.* 2006b, 27:2–16.

37. Weinberg RB. Apolipoprotein A-IV polymorphisms and diet-gene interactions. *Curr Opin Lipidol.* 2002, 13:125–134.

38. Lagrost L, Gambert P, Boquillon M, Lallemant C. Evidence for high density lipoproteins as the major apolipoprotein A-IV-containing fraction in normal human serum. *J Lipid Res.* 1989, 30:1525–1534.

39. Steinmetz A, Utermann G. Activation of lecithin: Cholesterol acyltransferase by human apolipoprotein A-IV. *J Biol Chem.* 1985, 260:2258–2264.

40. Chen CH, Albers JJ. Activation of lecithin: Cholesterol acyltransferase by apolipoproteins E-2, E-3, and A-IV isolated from human plasma. *Biochim Biophys Acta.* 1985, 836:279–285.

41. Main LA, Ohnishi T, Yokoyama S. Activation of human plasma cholesteryl ester transfer protein by human apolipoprotein A-IV. *Biochim Biophys Acta.* 1996, 1300:17–24.

42. Goldberg IJ, Scheraldi CA, Yacoub LK, Saxena U, Bisgaier CL. Lipoprotein ApoC-II activation of lipoprotein lipase. Modulation by apolipoprotein A-IV. *J Biol Chem.* 1990, 265:4266–4272.

43. Warner MM, Guo J, Zhao Y. The relationship between plasma apolipoprotein A-IV levels and coronary heart disease. *Chin Med J (Engl).* 2001, 114:275–279.

44. Wong WM, Hawe E, Li LK et al. Apolipoprotein AIV gene variant S347 is associated with increased risk of coronary heart disease and lower plasma apolipoprotein AIV levels. *Circ Res.* 2003, 92:969–975.
45. Kronenberg F, Stuhlinger M, Trenkwalder E et al. Low apolipoprotein A-IV plasma concentrations in men with coronary artery disease. *J Am Coll Cardiol.* 2000, 36:751–757.
46. Tenkanen H, Lukka M, Jauhiainen M, Metso J, Baumann M, Peltonen L, Ehnholm C. The mutation causing the common apolipoprotein A-IV polymorphism is a glutamine to histidine substitution of amino acid 360. *Arterioscler Thromb.* 1991, 11:851–856.
47. Menzel HJ, Boerwinkle E, Schrangl-Will S, Utermann G. Human apolipoprotein A-IV polymorphism: Frequency and effect on lipid and lipoprotein levels. *Hum Genet.* 1988, 79:368–372.
48. Weinberg RB. Apolipoprotein A-IV-2 allele: Association of its worldwide distribution with adult persistence of lactase and speculation on its function and origin. *Genet Epidemiol.* 1999, 17:285–297.
49. Kamboh MI, Ferrell RE. Genetic studies of human apolipoproteins. XV. An overview of IEF immunoblotting methods to screen apolipoprotein polymorphisms. *Hum Hered.* 1990, 40:193–207.
50. Sepehrnia B, Kamboh MI, Adams-Campbell LL, Nwankwo M, Ferrell RE. Genetic studies of human apolipoproteins. VII. Population distribution of polymorphisms of apolipoproteins A-I, A-II, A-IV, C-II, E, and H in Nigeria. *Am J Hum Genet.* 1988, 43:847–853.
51. Bai H, Saku K, Liu R, Oribe Y, Yamamoto K, Arakawa K. Polymorphism of the apolipoprotein A-IV gene and its significance in lipid metabolism and coronary heart disease in a Japanese population. *Eur J Clin Invest.* 1996, 26:1115–1124.
52. Saha N, Wang G, Vasisht S, Kamboh MI. Influence of two apo A4 polymorphisms at codons 347 and 360 on nonfasting plasma lipoprotein-lipids and apolipoproteins in Asian Indians. *Atherosclerosis.* 1997, 131:249–255.
53. Wang GQ, DiPietro M, Roeder K et al. Cladistic analysis of human apolipoprotein a4 polymorphisms in relation to quantitative plasma lipid risk factors of coronary heart disease. *Ann Hum Genet.* 2003, 67:107–124.
54. Yang CY, Gu ZW, Chong IS et al. The primary structure of human apolipoprotein A-IV. *Biochim Biophys Acta.* 1989, 1002:231–237.
55. Kamboh MI, Hamman RF, Ferrell RE. Two common polymorphisms in the APO A-IV coding gene: Their evolution and linkage disequilibrium. *Genet Epidemiol.* 1992, 9:305–315.
56. Zaiou M, Visvikis S, Gueguen R, Parra HJ, Fruchart JC, Siest G. DNA polymorphisms of human apolipoprotein A-IV gene: Frequency and effects on lipid, lipoprotein and apolipoprotein levels in a French population. *Clin Genet.* 1994, 46:248–254.
57. Groenendijk M, De Bruin TW, Dallinga-Thie GM. Two polymorphisms in the apo A-IV gene and familial combined hyperlipidemia. *Atherosclerosis.* 2001, 158:369–76.
58. Hockey KJ, Anderson RA, Cook VR, Hantgan RR, Weinberg RB. Effect of the apolipoprotein A-IV Q360H polymorphism on postprandial plasma triglyceride clearance. *J Lipid Res.* 2001, 42:211–217.
59. Ostos MA, Lopez-Miranda J, Ordovas JM et al. Dietary fat clearance is modulated by genetic variation in apolipoprotein A-IV gene locus. *J Lipid Res.* 1998, 39:2493–2500.
60. Miltiadous G, Hatzivassiliou M, Bashiardes E, Bairaktari E, Cariolou MA, Elisaf M. Genetic polymorphisms of the apolipoprotein A-IV in a Greek population and their relation to plasma lipid and lipoprotein levels. *Clin Genet.* 2002, 62:208–213.

61. Ganan A, Corella D, Guillen M, Ordovas JM, Pocovi M. Frequencies of apolipoprotein A4 gene polymorphisms and association with serum lipid concentrations in two healthy Spanish populations. *Hum Biol.* 2004, 76:253–266.
62. de Knijff P, Rosseneu M, Beisiegel U, de Keersgieter W, Frants RR, Havekes LM. Apolipoprotein A-IV polymorphism and its effect on plasma lipid and apolipoprotein concentrations. *J Lipid Res.* 1988, 1621–1627.
63. von Eckardstein A, Funke H, Schulte M, Erren M, Schulte H, Assmann G. Nonsynonymous polymorphic sites in the apolipoprotein (apo) A-IV gene are associated with changes in the concentration of apo B- and apo A-I-containing lipoproteins in a normal population. *Am J Hum Genet.* 1992, 50:1115–1128.
64. Carrejo MH, Sharrett R, Patsch W, Boerwinkle E. No association of apolipoprotein A-IV codon 347 and 360 variation with atherosclerosis and lipid transport in a sample of mixed hyperlipidemics. *Genet Epidemiol.* 1995, 12:371–380.
65. Larson IA, Ordovas JM, Sun Z et al. Effects of apolipoprotein A-IV genotype on glucose and plasma lipoprotein levels. *Clin Genet.* 2002, 61:430–436.
66. Cendorogo MS, Lahoz C, Martinez TL et al. Association of apo A-IV 360 (Gln→His) polymorphism with plasma lipids and lipoproteins: The Framingham Offspring Study. *Atherosclerosis.* 2005, 179:169–175.
67. Weinberg RB, Jordan MK, Steinmetz A. Distinctive structure and function of human apolipoprotein variant ApoA-IV-2. *J Biol Chem.* 1990, 265:18372–18378.
68. Ehnholm C, Tenkanen H, de Knijff P et al. Genetic polymorphism of apolipoprotein A-IV in five different regions of Europe. Relations to plasma lipoproteins and to history of myocardial infarction: The EARS study. European Atherosclerosis Research Study. *Atherosclerosis.* 1994, 107:229–238.
69. Rewers M, Kamboh MI, Hoag S, Shetterly SM, Ferrell RE, Hamman RF. ApoA-IV polymorphism associated with myocardial infarction in obese NIDDM patients. The San Luis Valley Diabetes Study. *Diabetes.* 1994, 43:1485–1489.
70. Herron KL, Lofgren IE, Adiconis X, Ordovas JM, Fernandez ML. Associations between plasma lipid parameters and APOC3 and APOA4 genotypes in a healthy population are independent of dietary cholesterol intake. *Atherosclerosis.* 2006, 184:113–120.
71. Tenkanen H, Koskinen P, Metso J et al. A novel polymorphism of apolipoprotein A-IV is the result of an asparagine to serine substitution at residue 127. *Biochim Biophys Acta.* 1992, 1138:27–33.
72. Wong WM, Stephens JW, Acharya J, Hurel SJ, Humphries SE, Talmud PJ. The APOA4 T347S variant is associated with reduced plasma TAOS in subjects with diabetes mellitus and cardiovascular disease. *J Lipid Res.* 2004, 45:1565–1571.
73. Qin X, Swertfeger DK, Zheng S, Hui DU, Tso P. Apolipoprotein AIV: A potent endogenous inhibitor of lipid oxidation. *Am J Physiol.* 1998, 274:H1836–1840.
74. Weinberg RB, Geissinger BW, Kasala K et al. Effect of apolipoprotein A-IV genotype and dietary fat on cholesterol absorption in humans. *J Lipid Res.* 2000, 41:2035–2041.
75. McCombs RJ, Marcadis DE, Ellis J, Weinberg RB. Attenuated hypercholesterolemic response to a high-cholesterol diet in subjects heterozygous for the apolipoprotein A-IV-2 allele. *N Engl J Med.* 1994, 331:706–710.
76. Jansen S, Lopez-Miranda J, Ordovas JM et al. Effect of 360His mutation in apolipoprotein A-IV on plasma HDL-cholesterol response to dietary fat. *J Lipid Res.* 1997, 38:1995–2002.
77. Wallace AJ, Humphries SE, Fisher RM, Mann JI, Chisholm A, Sutherland WH. Genetic factors associated with response of LDL subfractions to change in the nature of dietary fat. *Atherosclerosis.* 2000, 149:387–394.

78. Stan S, Delvin EE, Seidman E et al. Modulation of apo A-IV transcript levels and synthesis by n-3, n-6, and n-9 fatty acids in CACO-2 cells. *J Cell Biochem.* 1999, 75:73–81.
79. Kratz M, Wahrburg U, von Eckardstein A, Ezeh B, Assmann G, Kronenberg F. Dietary mono- and polyunsaturated fatty acids similarly increase plasma apolipoprotein A-IV concentrations in healthy men and women. *J Nutr.* 2003, 133:1821–1825.
80. Hajeer AH, Hutchinson IV. Influence of TNF-α gene polymorphisms on TNF-α production and disease. *Hum Immunol.* 2001, 62:1191–1199.
81. Bemelman MHA, van Tits LJH, Buurman WA. Tumor necrosis factor: Function, release and clearance. *Crit Rev Immunol.* 1996, 16:1–11
82. Libby P, Ridker PM. Novel inflammatory markers of coronary risk: Theory versus practice. *Circulation.* 1999, 100:1148–1150.
83. Danesh J, MBChb, Collins R, MBBS, Appleby P, Peto R. Association of fibrinogen, C-reactive protein, albumin, or leukocyte count with coronary heart disease: Meta-analyses of prospective studies. *JAMA.* 1998, 279:1477–1482.
84. Wilson AM, Ryan MC, Boyle AJ. The novel role of C-reactive protein in cardiovascular disease: Risk marker or pathogen. *Int. J Cardiology.* 2006, 106:291–297.
85. Bruunsgaard H, SkinhØJ P, Pedersen AN, Schroll M, Pedersen BK. Ageing, tumor necrosis factor-alpha (TNF-α) and atherosclerosis. *Clin Exp Immunol.* 2000, 121:255–260.
86. Skoog T, Dichtl W, Boquist S et al. Plasma tumor necrosis factor-α and early carotid atherosclerosis in healthy middle-aged men. *Eur Heart J.* 2002, 23:376–383.
87. Ridker PM, Rifai N, Pfeffer M, Sacks F, Lepage S, Braunwald E. Elevation of tumor necrosis factor-alpha and increased risk of recurrent coronary events after myocardial infarction. *Circulation.* 2000, 101:2149–2153.
88. Torre-Amione G, Kapadia S, Lee J et al. Tumor necrosis factor-α and tumor necrosis factor receptors in the failing human heart. *Circulation.* 1996, 93:704–711.
89. Barath P, Fishbein MC, Cao J et al. Detection and localization of TNF in human atheroma. *Am J Cardiol.* 1990, 65:297–302.
90. Kroeger KM, Carville KS, Abraham LJ. The −308 tumor necrosis factor-α promoter polymorphism effects transcription. *Molecular Immunol.* 1997, 34:391–399.
91. Wilson AM, Symons JA, McDowell TL, McDevitt HO, Duff GW. Effects of a polymorphism in the human tumor necrosis factor α promoter on transcriptional activation. *Proc. Natl Acad Sci USA.* 1997, 94:3195–3199.
92. Grimble RF, Howell WM, O'Reilly G et al. The ability of fish oil to suppress tumor necrosis factor α production by peripheral blood mononuclear cells in healthy men is associated with polymorphisms in genes that influence tumor necrosis factor α production. *Am J Clin Nutr.* 2002, 76:454–459.
93. Lakka HM, Lakka TA, Rankinen T et al. The TNF-α G-308A polymorphism is associated with C-reactive protein levels: The HERITAGE family study. *Vasc Harm.* 2006, 44:377–383.
94. The National Center for Biotechnology Information. <www.ncbi.nlm.nih.gov/snp.ref. cgi?rs=rs1800629> Accessed Jan. 14, 2007.
95. Herrmann S-M, Ricard S, Nicaud V et al. Polymorphisms of the tumor necrosis factor-α gene, coronary heart disease and obesity. *Eur J Clin Invest.* 1998, 28:59–66.
96. Keso T, Perola M, Laippala P et al. Polymorphisms within the tumor necrosis factor locus and prevalence of coronary artery disease in middle-aged men. *Atherosclerosis.* 2001, 154:691–697.
97. Padovani JC, Pazin-Filho A. Gene polymorphisms in the TNF locus and the risk of myocardial infarction. *Thrombosis Res.* 2000, 100:263–269.

98. Vendrell J, Fernandez-Real J-M, Gutierrez C, Zamora A, Simon I, Bardaji A, Ricart W, Richart C. A polymorphism in the promoter of the tumor necrosis factor-α gene (-308) is associated with coronary heart disease in type 2 diabetic patients. *Atherosclerosis.* 2003, 167:257–264.

99. Szalai C, Füst G, Duba J, Kramer J, Romics L, Prohászka Z, Császár A. Association of polymorphisms and allelic combinations in the tumor necrosis factor-α-complement MHC region with coronary artery disease. *J Med Genet.* 2002, 39:46–51.

100. Kang J-H, Sung M-K, Kawada T et al. Soybean saponins suppress the release of proinflammatory mediators by LPS-stimulated peritoneal macrophages. *Cancer Lett.* 2005, 230:219–227.

101. Horrigan LA, Kelly JP, Connor TJ. Caffeine suppresses TNF-α production via activation of the cyclic AMP/protein kinase A pathway. *Int Immunopharmacol.* 2004, 4:1409–1417.

CHAPTER **10**

Development of a Botanical Combination Product for Allergy Symptoms

Marc Lemay, David Fast, Yumei Lin, Charen Buyce, and Lisa Rozga

CONTENTS

INTRODUCTION

Allergy prevalence has increased over the past few decades,[1] and there is accumulating evidence that botanicals may be useful for the associated symptoms.[2–4] In order to commercialize a botanical dietary supplement to support clear nasal passages, we used an approach combining biological and clinical techniques. Botanical compounds with possible anti-allergic action that also met cost, availability, and global regulatory hurdles were screened in bioassays for anti-allergic action, singly and in various combinations. A selection of these was then submitted to skin-patch testing with human volunteers. Results from skin patch testing were used to formulate a potentially effective botanical combination formula based on a benchmark of wheal-size reduction associated with a standard anti-allergy pharmaceutical. This botanical formula was then tested in a double-blind, placebo-controlled clinical study using the nasal allergen challenge model of anti-allergic action. This sequence of actions can be seen as a model for achieving market entry and general market competitiveness of innovative technologies and products in the dietary supplement field.

IN VITRO SCREENING OF BOTANICALS

Identification of Botanicals

Potential anti-allergy botanicals were first identified from the medical and ethnopharmacological literature, from botanical products currently marketed around the world for allergy symptoms, and from discussions with raw-material suppliers. This produced a list of about 70 plant dehydrates, concentrates, or extracts. The potential ingredients were submitted to bioassay screening and regulatory review to narrow the potential active ingredients.

Materials and Methods

Mediator Release Assays

The symptoms of allergy are ultimately mediated by soluble mediators secreted by mast cells or basophils. Botanicals were therefore screened *in vitro* for inhibition of the allergic reaction mediators histamine, leukotriene C4 (LTC4), and prostaglandin D2 (PGD2). Following overnight treatment of rat basophilic leukemia cells (RBL-2H3) with botanicals, the cells were sensitized with an immunoglobulin E (IgE) specific for 2,4-dinitrophenol (DNP). Degranulation was triggered by the addition of DNP-bovine serum albumin (DNP-BSA) to cross-link the receptor-bound IgE. Following addition of DNP-BSA, supernatants were collected at 2 hours to measure histamine levels, and at 24 hours to measure LTC4 and PGD2, using ELISA kits obtained from Cayman Chemical (Ann Arbor, Michigan). All botanical samples were tested at 1 µg/ml.

Results

The data in Figure 10.1 show results from histamine, LTC4, and PGD2 release assays for selected botanicals. Results shown are means of two to eight replicate experiments with standard errors of the means and represent the effect of botanicals

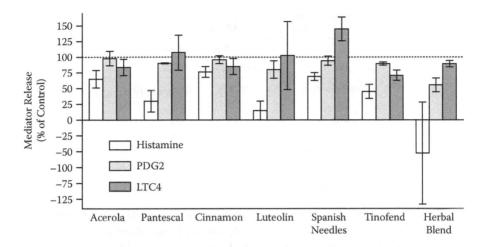

Figure 10.1 Effect of botanicals on allergy mediator release from stimulated cells.

on allergy mediator release from stimulated cells; for each mediator, "100%" represents the concentration of that mediator in the supernatant from stimulated cells. A result below 100% represents some inhibition of allergen mediator release, and below 0% represents inhibition below background levels (that is, in unstimulated cells).

The "Herbal Blend," composed of equal parts by weight of cinnamon bark extract (*Cinnamomum zeylanicum*), accrola fruit (*Mulpighia glabra*), and Spanish needles powder (*Bidens pilosa*), was one of the first combination formulas assayed. Surprisingly, it showed synergistic inhibition of histamine release: The sum of the inhibition of the three ingredients was 10.2% of control, whereas their combination inhibited histamine release to –52% (i.e., to below the concentration of histamine found in unstimulated cells).

Finally, the IC50 for inhibition of mediator release was calculated, based on the difference between background allergy mediator levels representing 0% and the total response induced by an IgE-allergen signal of 100%. For example, if histamine were found in the supernatant from unstimulated cells at 10 nM and from IgE-allergen-induced cells at 210 nM, the IC50 would be the concentration of botanical that reduced the amount of induced histamine (or PGD2 or LTC4) to 110 nm. The results in Table 10.1 show that Herbal Blend was a more potent inhibitor of histamine and PGD2 release than either of its components taken individually.

Discussion

A series of bioassays was utilized to screen a variety of single and combination botanical compounds for anti-allergy action *in vitro*. A combination of three ingredients—Herbal Blend—showed apparent synergistic inhibition of histamine. However, *in vitro* efficacy against allergic mediators does not ensure effectiveness in native disease—that is, in allergy sufferers in daily life. In addition, the commercial

Table 10.1   IC50 Values for Selected Botanicals
in Stimulated RBL-2H3 Cells[a]

| | Allergy Mediator | | |
Sample	Histamine	PGD2	LTC4
Herbal blend	0.005	5	10
Luteolin	0.05	15	0.05
Tinofend	0.1	>15	2
Acerola extract	1	>15	10
Cinnamon extract	>2	15	15
Spanish needles	>2	15	10

[a] Micrograms per milliliter.

prospects of a botanical product depend upon many more factors than just effectiveness. Bioassay results were thus evaluated with an ingredient selection matrix, which ranked botanicals on several weighted factors, each of which could affect the eventual product's commercial prospects for good or ill. Each of the factors shown in Table 10.2 has three rankings ordered from worst to best. For example, a botanical that had only anecdotal or historical evidence of efficacy for allergy symptoms would be ranked lower than one that had been shown efficacious in at least one controlled clinical study. Timing was also an issue, predicating higher ratings for a product that could be launched before, rather than after, the arrival of the spring allergy season. As well, botanicals that could be grown in-house, or "vertically integrated," thus allowing production and quality control from the seed to the finished product, were weighted more favorably than ingredients that could not.

Botanicals deemed acceptable by both bioassay testing and the matrix were submitted to a skin patch dose–response study for further refinement of the efficacy rating in the ingredient selection matrix. These botanicals included Spanish needles (*Bidens pilosa*) powder[5,6]; Perilla seed (*Perilla frutescens*) extract enriched for luteolin[7,8]; cinnamon bark (*Cinnamomum zeylanicum*) extract[9]; acerola fruit (*Malpighia glabra*) extract[10,11]; Pantescal®, a dietary supplement marketed in Italy containing *Capparis spinosa, Olea europeae, Glycyrrhiza glabra, Chamomilla matricaria, Ribes nigrae*, and *Panax ginseng*; Tinofend®, a commercial extract of *Tinospora cordifolia*[12]; luteolin[13]; and a novel combination of acerola extract, Spanish needles powder, and cinnamon extract (Herbal Blend; currently marketed in the United States as ClearGuard™).

SKIN PATCH DOSE–RESPONSE STUDY

Materials and Methods

A 4-week, single-blind, randomized, parallel-groups, dose–response study was conducted to test botanicals for allergy as measured by a skin patch test (wheal-and-flare reaction). The study was approved by an independent review board, informed consent was obtained before any screening or study measures, and the study was

Table 10.2   Ingredient Selection Matrix

Efficacy	Availability
• Only anecdotal evidence or historical usage • *In vitro* testing or uncontrolled clinical study • Randomized, double-blind, placebo-controlled clinical study	• Known supply shortages or price instability • Single supplier, with price increases possible • Multiple suppliers, costs stable

Cost

Marketing

Cost	Marketing
• Above target • At target • Below target	• No real differentiation, no clinical studies • Some differentiation, some uncontrolled clinical studies • Unique and differentiated, and clinically tested

Safety	Vertical Integration Potential
• Clinical data showing adverse events • Some animal studies with adverse events • Literature shows no positive or negative information on safety • Literature supports safe human use	• No possible integration • Grower can be certified • Can be vertically integrated

Technical Regulations	Legal Issues
• Product would be classified as a drug in one out of three key markets • Needs approval in two of three key markets • Acceptable in three key markets	• Not cleared in all target markets • Cleared in United States • Cleared in all target markets

Timing	Exclusivity/Patentability
• Launch after March 2006 • Launch in March 2006 • Launch before March 2006	• No exclusivity or patentability • Exclusivity in multilevel marketing channel or patentable in some markets • Exclusive in all channels and patentable in all target markets

conducted in accordance with the Helsinki Declaration. Subjects had to be from 18 to 65 years of age, be generally healthy, nonsmoking, and exhibit an allergic wheal-and-flare response to at least one of the following allergens administered in a screening skin patch test: timothy grass, sage, olive tree, sycamore tree, or elm tree pollens. A total of 24 male and female subjects (6 subjects per treatment) from the local (Los Angeles, California) area enrolled in the study. Following randomization, subjects were given test products to be taken three times a day by mouth (one or two capsules, depending on dose) with a meal. All products were packed in identical white capsules packed with an inert carrier, microcrystalline cellulose, as needed to ensure uniform weight. Three different treatment doses—"low," "medium," and "high"— were tested and skin-patch tests were performed in triplicate for each subject before the study and after 1 week of dosing at each dose. The order of dosing was from low to high in each subject, with no washout period between treatments. Four botanicals (combinations and single-ingredient formulations) were evaluated in all. Table 10.3 summarizes the dosing and composition of each tested botanical.

Table 10.3   Summary of Tested Botanicals and Dosages

| Botanical | Dosing Presentation[a] | | |
	Low Dose	Medium Dose	High Dose
Herbal blend (equal-weight combination of Spanish needles [*Bidens pilosa*] powder, acerola [*Malpighia glabra*] extract, and cinnamon [*Cinnamomum zeylanicum*] extract)	90 mg/dose in one capsule	135 mg/dose in one capsule	180 mg dose in one capsule
Pantescal® (*Capparis spinosa, Olea europeae, Glycyrrhiza glabra, Chamomilla matricaria, Ribes nigrae,* and *Panax ginseng*)	110 mg/dose in two capsules	220 mg/dose in two capsules	330 mg/dose in two capsules
Perilla frutescens (perilla leaf) extract enriched for luteolin	45 mg/dose in one capsule	60 mg/dose in one capsule	75 mg/dose in one capsule
Tinosporia cordifolia extract (TinoFend®)	100 mg/dose in two capsules	200 mg/dose in two capsules	300 mg/dose in two capsules

[a] All doses were three times a day for 1 week.

During the skin-prick test subjects were exposed to timothy grass, sage, olive tree, sycamore tree, and elm tree pollens on the surface of the forearm. A disposable hypodermic needle was passed through the allergen and inserted into the epidermal surface with the needle tip.[14,15] Subjects were also exposed to saline solution (as blank) and histamine (as positive control). The allergy reaction was measured 15 minutes after applying the allergens to the skin. A physician was present at all times in case of anaphylactic shock. Standard blood chemistries, hematology, and urinalysis were also performed before the study and at the end of each week's dosing, and adverse events were monitored.

Results

The allergens produced wheals 4–8 mm in diameter. Flares were not measured because of inconsistent appearance (some subjects had no flares, but all subjects had some wheal reaction). The wheal was measured by adhesive tape applied to the forearm, which when removed retained the outline of the wheal. The longest and shortest wheal diameters were averaged and these values were used to compare allergen reaction before and after treatment with the various botanicals and doses.

Data in Table 10.4 are shown as unadjusted allergen response data (that is, without reference to the saline condition) because of inconsistent response to histamine as the positive control, and large baseline between- and within-groups variability. Results for Herbal Blend showed a trend toward a dose–response effect (Figure 10.2). No significant adverse experiences were reported and results of serum chemistries, hematology, and urinalysis were not statistically different before and after treatment from all groups.

Table 10.4   Effect of Botanicals on Wheal Sizes[a]

Botanical	Low Dose	Medium Dose	High Dose
Herbal Blend	7.6 ± 3.4	6.5 ± 2.0	6.4 ± 3.0
Pantescal	5.9 ± 1.9	6.0 ± 1.0	5.8 ± 2.3
Perilla frutescens (perilla leaf) extract enriched for luteolin	7.4 + 2.9	5.8 ± 1.2	7.3 ± 2.7
Tinosporia cordifolia extract	7.0 ± 2.2	6.3 ± 1.0	7.4 ± 1.5

[a] Mean size in milimeters ± standard deviation.

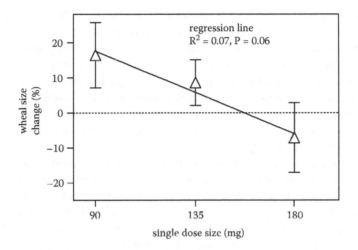

Figure 10.2   Wheal size change by Herbal Blend dose (means of replicate experiments ± SEM).

Discussion

The three different doses used in this study were estimated from concentrations shown to be effective against at least one allergy mediator *in vitro*. However, there is a large degree of uncertainty in such estimates based on the unknown bioavailability of the various active molecules in the botanicals. One way to reduce the uncertainty of the dose calculation is to relate the skin-patch results to similar results obtained from a well-known allergy drug. Loratadine is known to produce a 40% reduction in wheal size[15]; using this as a benchmark, by extrapolation one can calculate* that a dose of 315 mg of Herbal Blend would produce a 40% reduction in wheal size. However, the skin patch tests do not, any more than bioassays, ensure effectiveness in native disease. Therefore, after an evaluation of the safety and toxicology of

---

* The linear regression equation is $y = -0.26\,x + 41.13$.

these ingredients, and after consideration of uncertain bioavailability, Herbal Blend was formulated to contain 450 mg of the equal-weight mixture of cinnamon extract, acerola extract, and Spanish needles powder, and tested in a clinical study with a nasal allergen challenge.

NASAL ALLERGEN CHALLENGE CLINICAL STUDY

Material and Methods

Subjects for this randomized, double-blind, cross-over study were 20 otherwise healthy, adult, self-described allergy sufferers, currently asymptotic, recruited by the Allergy Research Foundation (Los Angeles, California). This study was approved by Coast Independent Review Board, and informed consent was obtained from all subjects. Only subjects who first tested positive for allergic reaction to allergen extracts in a skin-prick test were included. During the skin-prick test, subjects were exposed to pollen from timothy grass, sage, olive tree, sycamore tree, and elm tree, or animal-dander extract, producing a wheal-and-flare cutaneous reaction, which was measured 15 minutes after allergen challenge.

Subjects were assigned to receive loratadine (10 mg qd), Herbal Blend (450 mg tid), or placebo (tid) for 2 days before receiving a nasal allergen challenge (NAC). All tablets were coated the same color and all subjects took the same number of tablets (two tablets, three times a day) in a combination of active product or placebo as necessary to maintain blinding. The NACs were performed with diluent (NaCl, 0.9%, albumin, 0.3%) followed by increasing concentration of allergen challenge solution (50, 250, 1250, and 6250 allergy units [AUs])[16] administered at intervals (two sprays per nostril) over about 2 hours. Ten minutes after each challenge, nasal symptoms were measured with an 11-point nasal symptom score (NSS) scale as follows:

> sneezing (number of sneezes in 10 min): 3 or 4 = 1, greater than 5 = 2
> rhinorrhea: runny nose = 1, postnasal drip = 1, both = 3
> nasal blockage: breathes freely = 0, breathes with difficulty = 1, one nostril blocked =
>   2, both nostrils blocked = 3
> pruritus: nose = 1, palate or ear = 1
> conjunctivitis = 1

Total maximum score was 11.[17] Nasal lavage samples were also taken before and immediately after the nasal allergen challenge and analyzed for the allergic reaction and inflammatory mediators PGD2; leukotrienes C, T, and E4; and tryptase.

After the NAC, subjects were free to go and continued rating their symptoms every 2 hours for an 8-hour follow-up period using the NSS scale. Subjects also continued dosing during that 8-hour follow-up. Following a 3-day washout, the procedure was repeated, until all subjects had tried all products.

The primary outcome analysis was a series of one-tailed paired t-tests to compare each subject's placebo measurement to his or her treatment measurement at each time point as well as overall, using the sum of NSS for the 8-hour period after the NAC, as well as area under the NSS curve for the entire period including the NAC. All results are reported as means ± standard errors of the means.

Results

Twenty subjects (nine men and 11 women) with a mean age of 38 years took part in this study. Of those subjects, 17 completed all treatments (placebo, loratadine, and Herbal Blend); three subjects who were unable to attend all test sessions were excluded from pair-wise analyses on a per-comparison basis. The demographic variables for subjects in this study are listed in Table 10.5.

Table 10.5   Demographic Characteristics of the Study Population

No. of subjects	20
Mean age (SD) (y)	38.2 (3.34)
Mean height (SD) (in)	64.7 (3.56)
Mean weight (SD) (lb)	153.5 (31.57)
Sex (%):	
Male	45
Female	55

Early-Phase Response

During the NAC, loratadine was associated with significantly fewer symptoms than placebo at the highest dose of allergen (6250 AUs) ($P = 0.04$, $t = 1.83$, df = 19) as well as overall, expressed as the sum of nasal symptom scores experienced over the NAC ($P = 0.04$, $t = 1.83$, df = 19). During the NAC, there were no statistically significant differences between Herbal Blend and placebo at any time point (Figure 10.3).

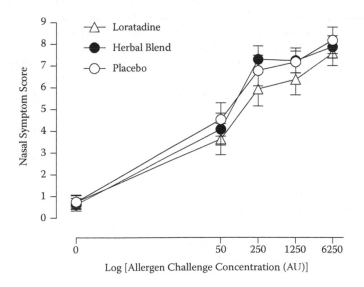

Figure 10.3   Early-phase nasal symptom scores.

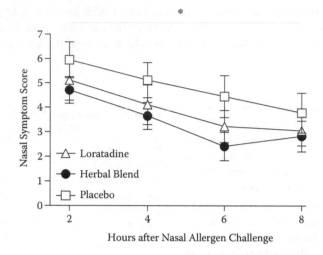

Figure 10.4 Nasal symptom scores during late-phase response. * = P = 0.04 for Herbal Blend and placebo areas over NSS curves; ** = P = 0.007 Herbal Blend versus placebo at 6 h.

Late-Phase Response

After the NAC, subjects taking Herbal Blend continued dosing following a tid schedule (i.e., two more doses), and subjects in the other treatment conditions continued taking placebo while rating their nasal symptoms with the NSS scale every 2 hours for 8 hours. During this late phase (that is, at 2, 4, 6, and 8 hours after the NAC), loratadine led to significantly fewer NSSs than placebo at 6 hours (P = 0.01, t = 2.57, df = 17) and overall (P = 0.04, t = 1.82, df = 17). Herbal Blend also led to significantly fewer NSSs than placebo at 6 hours (P = 0.007, t = 2.74, df = 16) and overall (P = 0.04, t = 1.86, df = 16). There were also trends toward significantly fewer symptoms than placebo at 4 hours for loratadine (P = 0.09, t = 1.73, df = 17) and at 2 and 4 hours for Herbal Blend (P = 0.09, t = 1.39, df = 16, and P = 0.05, t = 1.71, df = 16, respectively) (Figure 10.4).

Analysis of NSS areas over the curve, a clinically relevant measure of total product effect over the 8-hour period following the NAC, showed that loratadine and Herbal Blend were not significantly different from each other (P = 0.28, t = –0.6, df = 16) and that both were significantly better than placebo (P = 0.03, t = 1.96, df = 17 for loratadine, and P = 0.03, t = 2.04, df = 16 for Herbal Blend) (Figure 10.5).

Loratadine led to significantly fewer sneezes per 2-hour period compared to placebo at 6 hours (P = 0.02, t = 2.22, df =16) and 8 hours, (P = 0.03, t = 1.89, df = 16) as well as overall (P = 0.04, t = 1.79, df = 16), after the NAC. Herbal Blend reduced sneezing compared to placebo at 6 hours (P = 0.04, t = 1.93, df = 16) as well as overall (P = 0.04, t = 1.76, df = 16), with a trend toward significance at 2 and 4 hours (Figure 10.6).

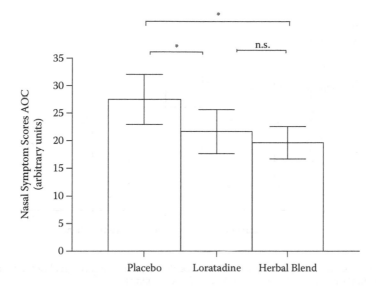

Figure 10.5   Nasal symptom scores areas over the curve by treatment. * = P < 0.05.

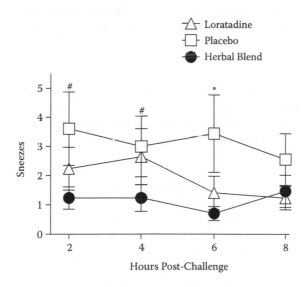

Figure 10.6   Objective sneeze counts during late phase (2–8 h after nasal challenge). # and
* = P < 0.10 and 0.05, respectively, Herbal Blend versus placebo.

Analysis of allergic mediators in nasal fluid before and immediately after the
NAC showed that prostaglandin D2 concentration changes were significantly different from zero in the loratadine (two-tailed Wilcoxon signed rank test P = 0.006) and

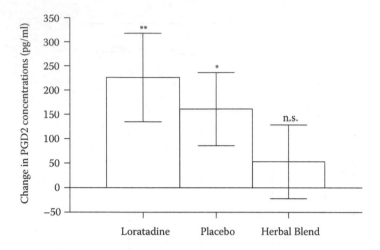

Figure 10.7 Change in prostaglandin D2 concentrations following nasal challenge, by treatment. Means with SE ** = P < 0.01, * = P < 0.05, nonsignificant.

placebo (two-tailed Wilcoxon signed rank test P = 0.04) treatment conditions, but not in the Herbal Blend treatment condition (two-tailed Wilcoxon signed rank test P = 0.62) (Figure 10.7). Neither treatment significantly affected tryptase or leukotriene C4 release or inflammatory cell infiltration (data not shown).

Safety

Blood chemistries, hematology, and urinalysis were performed before and after each 3-day period of dosing. Review of laboratory findings as well as subjective adverse event reports revealed no untoward signs or symptoms associated with consumption of any of the products during this study.

DISCUSSION

Using a standard nasal allergen challenge model of allergy and anti-allergic action in a blinded, active- and placebo-controlled cross-over study, Herbal Blend was shown to have a significant anti-allergy action on three levels: subjective (nasal symptoms scores), objective (sneeze counts), and biochemical (nasal lavage assays of PGD2). The magnitude of the difference using the NSS scale was about 1.5 points on an 11-point scale. The smallest clinically meaningful difference in allergy treatment effects is about a 0.5 score step on a composite scale like the NSS.[18] Thus, the clinical results with Herbal Blend are clinically meaningful—a conclusion also supported by the comparison to loratadine, which was associated with symptom relief greater than placebo but not significantly different from Herbal Blend.

There are several limitations to this clinical study. The nasal allergen challenge model of anti-allergic action is difficult to generalize precisely to native disease. The bioassay screening data suggested a quick-acting antihistamine effect, which was not found in the clinical study, where effects were more suggestive of slower-acting anti-inflammatory action. The nasal lavage data were equivocal; there were significant rises in PGD2 nasal concentrations in the loratadine and placebo treatment conditions but not in the Herbal Blend condition. However, there were no significant intergroup differences.

The active ingredients on a molecular level are unknown, but there are indications in the literature that all three botanical ingredients can possess anti-allergic action:

Cinnamomum cassia, a species of cinnamon related to that found in Herbal Blend, inhibits complement-dependent allergic reaction by reducing immunological hemolysis, chemotactic migration of neutrophils, and the generation of chemotactic factors by mast cells in response to complement-activated serum.[9]

Acerola contains vitamin C, which is associated with lower risk of asthma,[19,20] and a regular use of vitamin C has been shown to reduce concentrations of histamine, a major allergic reaction and inflammatory mediator.[21,22]

Spanish needles have also been found to have anti-allergy action at the level of mast cells and other allergy mediators.[4] Spanish needles contains quercetin and ethyl caffeate, both of which have previously been shown to possess *in vitro* anti-inflammatory or anti-allergic mediator action.[23,74] Quercetin[5] has also been shown to stabilize mast cells and basophils, decrease leukotriene formation, and reduce release of histamine and other mediators.[24,25] Anti-inflammatory effects have been demonstrated in rats after receiving aqueous extracts of Spanish needles leaves and stems.[26,27] A related species, *Bidens parviflora,* has been reported to inhibit histamine release from rat mast cells *in vitro.*[6] Spanish needles have been shown to inhibit the inflammatory mediator nuclear transcription factor kappaB (NF-kappaB) and its downstream inflammatory mediators *in vitro.*[23]

Suppression of NF-kappaB has also been observed with a wide variety of phytochemicals found in common spices and food plants.[28] It is likely that the clinical anti-allergic action found in this clinical study is due to the combined activity of many phytochemicals in all three botanical ingredients.

These results have important clinical implications, not only in allergic rhinitis but also in many other diseases, including asthma, perennial rhinitis, and nasal polyposis. Both bioassay and nasal lavage data from a human clinical trial suggest Herbal Blend inhibits histamine and PGD2 release or synthesis. Ideally, the present bioassays using a rat basophilic cell line would need to be replicated using human mast cells. In addition, future clinical studies could evaluate PGD2 synthesis because the disconnect between histamine and PGD2 levels in the bioassays and nasal lavage data (the former suggesting strong inhibition of histamine and weak inhibition of PGD2, the latter the converse) suggests that the mechanism of action of Herbal Blend is more, or other, than simply preventing widespread mast cell degranulation.

In conclusion, a three-stage research program utilizing bioassays, skin-patch testing, and nasal allergen challenge testing, with each step closer to predicting actual human benefit, was successfully utilized to support the effectiveness of a dietary supplement for the support of clear nasal passages.

REFERENCES

1. Liu, A.H. Allergy and asthma prevention: The cup half full. *Allergy Asthma Proc,* 22(6), 333–336, 2001.
2. Meletis, C.D. Nutrient support to minimize the allergic cascade. *Altern Compl Ther,* 5,102–105, 1999.
3. Passalacqua, G., Bousquet, P.J., Carlsen, K.H., Kemp, J., Lockey, R.F., Niggemann, B., Pawankar, R., Price, D., and Bousquet, J. ARIA update: I—Systematic review of complementary and alternative medicine for rhinitis and asthma. *J Allergy Clin Immunol,* 117(5), 1054–1062, 2006.
4. Theoharides, T.C. and Bielory, L. Mast cells and mast cell mediators as targets of dietary supplements. *Ann Allergy Asthma Immunol,* 93(2 Suppl 1), S24–34, 2004.
5. Oliveira, F.Q., Andrade-Neto, V., Krettli, A.U., and Brandao, M.G. New evidences of antimalarial activity of *Bidens pilosa* roots extract correlated with polyacetylene and flavonoids. *J Ethnopharmacol,* 93(1), 39–42, 2004.
6. Wang, N., Yao, X., Ishii, R., and Kitanaka, S. Antiallergic agents from natural sources. 3. Structures and inhibitory effects on nitric oxide production and histamine release of five novel polyacetylene glucosides from *Bidens parviflora* Willd. *Chem Pharm Bull (Tokyo),* 49(8), 938–942, 2001.
7. Takano, H., Osakabe, N., Sanbongi, C., Yanagisawa, R., Inoue, K., Yasuda, A., Natsume, M., Baba, S., Ichiishi, E., and Yoshikawa, T. Extract of *Perilla frutescens* enriched for rosmarinic acid, a polyphenolic phytochemical, inhibits seasonal allergic rhinoconjunctivitis in humans. *Exp Biol Med (Maywood),* 229(3), 247–254, 2004.
8. Makino, T., Furuta, Y., Wakushima, H., Fujii, H., Saito, K., and Kano, Y. Anti-allergic effect of *Perilla frutescens* and its active constituents. *Phytother Res,* 17(3), 240–243, 2003.
9. Nagai, H., Shimazawa, T., Matsuura, N., and Koda, A. Immunopharmacological studies of the aqueous extract of *Cinnamomum cassia* (CCAq). I. Anti-allergic action. *Jpn J Pharmacol,* 32(5), 813–822, 1982.
10. Itoo, S., Aiba, M., and Ishihata, K. Comparison of ascorbic acid content in acerola fruit from different production regions depend on degree of maturity, and its stability by processing. *Nippon Shokuhin Kogyo Gakkaishi,* 37, 726–729, 1990.
11. Ford, E.S., Mannino, D.M., and Redd, S.C. Serum antioxidant concentrations among U.S. adults with self-reported asthma. *J Asthma,* 41,179–87, 2004.
12. Badar, V.A., Thawani, V.R., Wakode, P.T., Shrivastava, M.P., Gharpure, K.J., Hingorani, L.L., and Khiyani, R.M. Efficacy of *Tinospora cordifolia* in allergic rhinitis. *J Ethnopharmacol,* Jan 15, 96(3):445–449, 2005. Epub 2004 Nov 23.
13. Das, M., Ram, A., and Ghosh, B. Luteolin alleviates bronchoconstriction and airway hyperreactivity in ovalbumin sensitized mice. *Inflamm Res,* 52(3), 101–106, 2003.
14. Nelson, H. S., Knoetzer, J., and Bucher, B. Effect of distance between sites and region of the body on results of skin-prick tests. *J Allergy Clin Immunol,* 97(2), 596–601, 1996.
15. Roongapinun, S., Wajajamreon, S., and Fooanant, S. Comparative efficacy of wheal-and-flare suppression among various nonsedating antihistamines and the pharmacologic insights to their efficacy. *J Med Assoc Thai,* May, 87(5), 551–556, 2004.
16. Corren, J., Rachelefsky, G., Spector, S., Schanker, H., Siegel, S., Holton, D., Karcher, K., and Travers, S. Onset and duration of action of levocabastine nasal spray in atopic patients under nasal challenge conditions. *J Allergy Clin Immunol,* 103(4), 574–580, 1999.

17. Bousquet, J., Lebel, B., Chanal, I., Morel, A., and Michel, F. B. Antiallergic activity of H1-receptor antagonists assessed by nasal challenge. *J Allergy Clin Immunol,* 82(5 Pt 1), 881–887, 1988.
18. Akerlund, A., Andersson, M., Leflein, J., Lildholdt, T., and Mygind, N. Clinical trial design, nasal allergen challenge models, and considerations of relevance to pediatrics, nasal polyposis, and different classes of medication. *J Allergy Clin Immunol,* 115, S460–482, 2005.
19. Harik-Khan, R.I., Muller, D.C., and Wise, R.A. Serum vitamin levels and the risk of asthma in children. *Am J Epidemiol,* 159, 351–357, 2004.
20. Olusi, S.O., Ojutiku, O.O., Jessop, W.J., and Iboko, M.I. Plasma and white blood cell ascorbic acid concentrations in patients with bronchial asthma. *Clin Chim Acta,* 92,161–166, 1979.
21. Johnston, C.S., Martin, L.J., and Cai, X. Antihistamine effect of supplemental ascorbic acid and neutrophil chemotaxis. *J Am Coll Nutr,* 11, 172–176, 1992.
22. Pearce, F. L., Befus, A. D., and Bienenstock, J. Mucosal mast cells. III. Effect of quercetin and other flavonoids on antigen-induced histamine secretion from rat intestinal mast cells. *J Allergy Clin Immunol,* 73(6), 819–823, 1984.
23. Chiang, Y.M., Lo, C.P., Chen, Y.P., Wang, S.Y., Yang, N.S., Kuo, Y.H., and Shyur, L.F. Ethyl caffeate suppresses NF-kappaB activation and its downstream inflammatory mediators, iNOS, COX-2, and PGE2 *in vitro* or in mouse skin. *Br J Pharmacol,* 146(3), 352–363, 2005.
24. Chiang, Y.M., Chuang, D.Y., Wang, S.Y., Kuo, Y.H., Tsai, P.W., and Shyur, L.F. Metabolite profiling and chemopreventive bioactivity of plant extracts from *Bidens pilosa*. *J Ethnopharmacol,* 95(2–3), 409–419, 2004.
25. Yoshimoto, T., Furukawa, M., Yamamoto, S., Horie, T., and Watanabe-Kohno, S. Flavonoids: Potent inhibitors of arachidonate 5-lipoxygenase. *Biochem Biophys Res Commun,* 116, 612–618, 1983.
26. Chih, H.W., Lin, C.C., and Tang, K.S. Anti-inflammatory activity of Taiwan folk medicine "ham-hong-chho" in rats. *Am J Chin Med,* 23, 273–278, 1995.
27. Jager, A.K., Hutchings, A., and van Staden, J. Screening of Zulu medicinal plants for prostaglandin-synthesis inhibitors. *J Ethnopharmacol,* 52, 95–100, 1996.
28. Aggarwal, B.B. and Shishodia, S. Suppression of the nuclear factor-kappaB activation pathway by spice-derived phytochemicals: Reasoning for seasoning. *Ann NY Acad Sci,* Dec, 1030, 434–41, 2004.

CHAPTER 11

Genotype-Selective Inhibition of IL-1 by Botanicals
A Nutrigenetics Proof of Principle

R. Keith Randolph

CONTENTS

ABSTRACT

Emerging research now suggests that a number of prevalent, well characterized single nucleotide polymorphisms (SNPs) interact with environmental factors to influence a range of physiological parameters, including lipid metabolism, cognitive function, bone mineral density, inflammatory response, and others. These gene–environment interactions conceptually present an opportunity to customize or personalize nutritional and lifestyle interventions that should favorably influence the impact of polymorphisms and balance an individual's physiology toward a more optimum function. Toward this end, we set out to identify botanicals to balance interleukin IL-1 overexpression in IL1 composite genotyped individuals overexpressing IL-1. This chapter summarizes the development program strategy and results obtained in a pilot clinical trial. Results from the pilot clinical trial lend directional evidence that nutrigenetic interventions are feasible.

INTRODUCTION

The beneficial impact of the application of nutrigenetic principles is that genetic information may be used to guide individuals to better nutrition and lifestyle choices. This premise assumes that some individuals will have health benefits from consumption of certain nutrients and other individuals will have either less benefit or adverse reactions. In an effort to develop practical consumer applications of nutrigenetics, we focused on the role of genetic variations in key inflammatory mechanisms as a target for nutrient modulation.

Inflammation is now well recognized as a significant contributor to the pathogenesis of cardiovascular disease as well as a number of other chronic degenerative conditions (Figure 11.1) [1–6]. The genes encoding the pro-inflammatory cytokines IL-1α and IL-1β are among the first activated in the course of an inflammatory response. Recent studies have shown that IL1 gene variations alter gene expression, are associated with higher levels of IL-1β and other inflammatory mediators, and are associated with an increased risk of early myocardial infarction (MI) [7–11].

The IL1 genotypes that constitute the IL1[Pos] group in this study have been shown to increase the risk of early myocardial infarction and increase the expression of IL-1β [4,11].

This proof-of-concept development effort was designed to determine whether individuals with the genetic variations that predispose them to overexpression of IL-1 and premature heart disease could be modulated by means of botanicals that were selected for this specific IL-1 target. In this work we used cell-based models to screen botanicals that inhibited IL-1β. Healthy subjects were selected with elevated C-reactive protein (CRP) and were stratified into genetic groups based on being either positive (IL1[Pos]) or negative (IL1[Neg]) for the IL1 gene variations associated with overexpression of IL-1 and increased risk for early cardiovascular events. IL1[Pos] and IL1[Neg] subjects were then randomized to various candidate botanical extracts selected from the screening assays. In this study, consumption of the botanicals mixture for 4 weeks inhibited IL1 gene expression significantly in IL1[Pos] subjects, but there was less effect in IL1[Neg] subjects. This represents one of a few prospective clinical proofs that selected botanicals can differentially influence physiological mechanisms based on genetic variations.

METHODS OVERVIEW

The goal of the research program was to identify and clinically test botanicals directed at reducing selected inflammatory mediators in healthy individuals who have

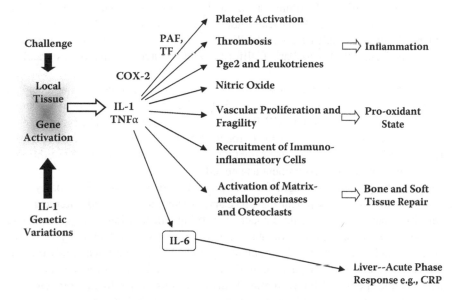

Variations in Upstream Response Genes Influence Downstream
Events Sufficiently to Alter Clinical Expression of Disease

Figure 11.1 Variations in upstream response genes influence downstream events sufficiently to alter clinical expression of disease.

genetic variations associated with overexpression of IL-1 and with increased risk for early cardiovascular events. The overview of the program is shown in Table 11.1.

Participant Database

A participant database was created under an Independent Review Board (IRB)-approved protocol (Western IRB, Olympia, Washington) (Table 11.1, activity 1). The ata collection process began in October 2003 and continued through April 2005 at

Table 11.1 Overview of the Program

Activity	Test System	Key Outcomes
1. Recruit volunteers who met entrance requirements	Establishing a clinical genotyped database	Adequate number of healthy subjects with CRP = 2–10 mg/L and stratified by IL1 composite genotype
2. Screen botanical ingredients for inhibition of IL-1β production	Human monocyte cell lines stimulated *in vitro* with LPS	Select lead candidate botanicals based on IL-1 protein inhibitory dose$_{50}$ compared to untreated cultures
3. Pilot clinical evaluation of IL-1 Inhibitory lead candidate botanicals from activity 2	Clinical + laboratory assay of peripheral blood mononuclear cells (PBMCs), and plasma	IL1 gene expression in PBMCs and *ex vivo* IL-1 production in plasma from test subjects after 2-week dosing of candidate botanicals

eight research sites throughout the United States (Access Business Group, Buena Park, California; Alticor, Ada, Michigan; East Coast Clinical Research, Salisbury, Massachusetts; National Institute for Clinical Research, Los Angeles, California; Omega Medical Research, Warwick, Rhode Island; Providence Clinical Research, Burbank, California; Sall Research Medical Center, Bellflower, California; Southbay Pharma Research, Buena Park, California) and resulted in a database of healthy adults.

After providing informed consent under the approved protocol, all subjects had a fasting blood sample collected and completed the 38-question Personal Wellness Profile Concise Assessment Plus (Wellsource, Clacamas, Oregon). The blood sample was used for determination of plasma C-reactive protein level and DNA extraction to determine IL1 genotype. Aliquots of the blood samples were archived for additional genotyping or biomarker assessment as needed.

All resulting laboratory data for this project were sent to a third-party data manager (Ockham Development Group; Cary, North Carolina) and entered into a secured database containing no subject-identifying information. The sponsor had access only to the de-identified database for purposes such as data analysis, report generation, and identification of candidates by code for future clinical study recruitment. Recruitment from the participant database involved a decoding step not associated with the sponsor. All intervention trials were constrained by randomization to include equal numbers of different genotyped subjects such that genotype and other protected information were not revealed by recruitment inclusion/exclusion criteria.

IL1 Genotype Stratification of Subjects

DNA was extracted and genotyping was performed by Kimball Genetics Inc, Denver, Colorado. All genetic analyses were performed blinded to clinical data.

Single nucleotide polymorphisms were genotyped at two loci in the gene for IL-1β [IL1β (-511) C > T; and IL1β (+3954) C > T], and at one locus in the gene for IL-1α [IL1A (+4845) G > T]. The three IL1 SNPs were selected based on the following:

> IL1β (-511) allele C has been associated with increased expression of IL-1β protein and with increased risk for cardiovascular events [7].
> IL1β (+3954) allele T, either alone or in combination with IL1α (+4845) allele T, has been associated with increased levels of IL-1 and CRP [5–7,9].

Subjects were classified into two genotype groups. The first group, IL1[Pos], included composite genotypes with IL1 alleles that have been previously associated with overexpression of inflammatory mediators; the second group, IL1[Neg], included all other genotypes that had not been associated with overexpression of inflammatory mediators.

Subjects possessing one copy of allele 2 at the +4845 locus of the IL1α gene [IL1α (+4845) = 2.2] or one copy of allele 2 at the +4845 locus of the IL1α gene and at least one copy of allele 2 at the +3954 locus of the IL1β gene [IL1α (+4845) = 1.2 and IL1β (+3954) = 1.2 or 2.2], or one copy of allele 2 at the 2018 locus of the IL1RN gene, or no copies of allele 2 at any of the four loci tested were designated IL1^{Pos}. All other individuals were designated IL1^{Neg}.

Ingredient Screening for Inhibition of IL-1 Production

Screening involved evaluation of 220 candidate botanical ingredients *in vitro* for their ability to inhibit IL1β gene expression in human mononuclear cells (U937 and THP-1) that were stimulated with lipopolysaccharide (LPS) (Table 11.1, activity 2). The ingredient list was narrowed to twenty-six botanicals that had a 50% inhibitory concentration of ≤10 μg/ml in the *in vitro* IL-1 production assay. The potential IL-1 inhibitors were further narrowed to four botanicals (artichoke leaf extract, nettle root extract, olive fruit extract, and rose hips extract) based on criteria such as reliability of sourcing, purity, and others that might contribute to commercial potential.

Pilot Clinical Evaluation of Lead Candidates for Inhibition of IL1 Gene Expression and Production

The protocol for pilot evaluation of the four IL-1 inhibiting botanicals was approved by New England IRB (Wellesley, Massachusetts), and all subjects who participated in the study gave their informed consent (Table 11.1, activity 3). Study volunteers were recruited from the genotyped database described earlier. Fifty subjects, twenty-five of each IL1 genotype, were randomized equally across four botanical intervention arms or pentoxifylline, a drug that has been reported to reduce CRP levels. The trial was a double-blind, six-arm parallel, 2-week design. Each of the four botanicals was formulated into tablets and IL1^{Pos} and IL1^{Neg} subjects were dosed once daily for 2 weeks with one of the botanicals. Table 11.2 summarizes the four botanicals, markers, and dose per day administered during the pilot clinical trial.

Peripheral blood mononuclear cells (PBMCs) were collected from experimental subjects and evaluated for IL1β gene expression at baseline and after 2 weeks of dosing. In vivo IL1 gene expression was assessed in participants' blood cells using quantitative real-time polymerase chain reaction (PCR). To this end, total RNA was isolated from whole blood samples and reverse transcribed to cDNA. Real-time PCR was performed using fluorescent-labeled specific primers for IL1β. An absolute quantitation of IL1β mRNA was measured and expressed in terms of RNA concentration in the sample. In absolute quantitations, signal intensities representing the expression levels of the gene of interest were compared to a standard curve generated

Table 11.2   Botanicals, Markers and Daily Dose

Botanical	Markers	Dose/Day (mg)
Rose hips extract	Dehydro-ascorbate	1200
Blackberry powder	Chlorogenic acid	165
Blueberry powder	Anthocyanins	330
Grape vine extract	All-*trans*-resveratrol	40

by a concentration titration of an external standard, which was synthetic IL1β RNA in this study.

Plasma from subjects at baseline and after 2 weeks of dosing was also evaluated *ex vivo* for IL-1β protein release in THP-1 cells stimulated with LPS.

The *ex vivo* IL-1β production was measured prior to administration of study product on the day blood samples were taken. The participants' plasma was incubated with a THP-1 human mononuclear cell line *in vitro*. The cultured cells were then challenged with LPS, and the production of IL1β was evaluated by ELISA methodology.

RESULTS

There were no significant differences between any of the treatment groups at baseline between genotypes or for *in vivo* IL-1 gene expression, or ex vivo IL-1 production.

Of all four botanicals tested, only rose hips elicited a consistent effect on reducing *in vivo* IL1 gene expression and *ex vivo* IL-1 production. Moreover, this effect was observed only in IL1[Pos] individuals. No consistent effects in either genotype group or with the other botanicals were observed. For IL1[Pos] individuals consuming rose hips, IL-1 gene expression was reduced 46% on average relative to baseline, and *ex vivo* IL-1 production was reduced 32% in the same individuals. Owing to the small size of this pilot trial, statistical analyses were not performed.

Adverse Events

Test products were well tolerated with infrequent and minor adverse events. With regard to safety outcomes, hematologies and serum chemistries tracked throughout the intervention within two standard deviations of baseline values.

DISCUSSION

The randomized nutrigenetics clinical trial demonstrates that a botanical targeting IL-1 production and response reduced IL1 gene expression in healthy individuals carrying gene variations that are associated with overexpression of IL-1. The botanical extracts were selected from *in vitro* screens designed to assess modulation of IL-1β overexpression, the biological effect associated with the IL1[Pos] genotypes used in the clinical study. The clinical study population included healthy adults with CRP levels between 2 and 10 mg/L. These individuals were then stratified by IL1 composite genotype prior to randomization to the botanicals. We believe this pilot trial points to the clinical potential of nutrigenetics and supports the feasibility to develop a nutritional product to modulate directly the effects of a genetic variation.

The outcomes of this pilot trial led to the design and execution of a larger prospective intervention that evaluated multibotanical formulas based upon rose hips as a foundational ingredient. The results of this clinical trial have been published elsewhere [12].

ACKNOWLEDGMENTS

Thanks to Ken Kornman and John Rogus, Interleukin Genetics, Waltham, Massachusetts; and Haeri Roh-Schmidt, David Krempin, Audra J. Davies, and Kerry Grann, Nutrilite Health Institute, Buena Park, California.

REFERENCES

1 Dziedzic T. Systemic inflammatory markers and risk of dementia. *Am J Alzheimer's Dis Other Demen* 2006, 21(4): 258–262.
2. Ravaglia G, Forti P, Maioli F, Chiappelli M, Montesi F, Tumini E et al. Blood inflammatory markers and risk of dementia: The Conselice Study of Brain Aging. *Neurobiol Aging* 2007, 28(12):1810–1820.
3. Heneka MT, O'Banion MK. Inflammatory processes in Alzheimer's disease. *J Neuroimmunol* 2007, 184(1–2):69–91.
4. Kornman KS. Interleukin 1 genetics, inflammatory mechanisms, and nutrigenetic opportunities to modulate diseases of aging. *Am J Clin Nutr* 2006, 83(2):475S–483S.
5. Libby P. Inflammation and cardiovascular disease mechanisms. *Am J Clin Nutr* 2006, 83(2):456S–460S.
6. Ridker PM, Cannon CP, Morrow D, Rifai N, Rose LM, McCabe CH et al. C-reactive protein levels and outcomes after statin therapy. *N Engl J Med* 2005, 352(1):20–28.
7. Kirii H, Niwa T, Yamada Y, Wada H, Saito K, Iwakura Y et al. Lack of interleukin-1beta decreases the severity of atherosclerosis in ApoE-deficient mice. *Arterioscler Thromb Vasc Biol* 2003, 23(4):656–660.
8. Nicklin MJ, Barton JL, Nguyen M, FitzGerald MG, Duff GW, Kornman K. A sequence-based map of the nine genes of the human interleukin-1 cluster. *Genomics* 2002, 79(5): 718–725.
9. Isoda K, Sawada S, Ishigami N, Matsuki T, Miyazaki K, Kusuhara M et al. Lack of interleukin-1 receptor antagonist modulates plaque composition in apolipoprotein E-deficient mice. *Arterioscler Thromb Vasc Biol* 2004, 24(6):1068–1073.
10. Chen H, Wilkins LM, Aziz N, Cannings C, Wyllie DH, Bingle C et al. Single nucleotide polymorphisms in the human interleukin-1B gene affect transcription according to haplotype context. *Hum Mol Genet* 2006, 15(4):519–529.
11. Iacoviello L, Di Castelnuovo A, Gattone M, Pezzini A, Assanelli D, Lorenzet R et al. Polymorphisms of the interleukin-1beta gene affect the risk of myocardial infarction and ischemic stroke at young age and the response of mononuclear cells to stimulation *in vitro. Arterioscler Thromb Vasc Biol* 2005, 25(1):222–227.
12. Kornman, K, Rogus, J, Roh-Schmidt, HR, Krempin, D, Davies, AJ, Grann, K, Randolph, RK. IL-1 genotype-selective inhibition of inflammatory mediators by a botanical. *Nutrition* 2007, 23(11–12):844–852.

Index

A

Aβ peptides, 113
  black tea and, 113
  EC and, 113
  ECG and, 113
  EGC and, 113
  EGCG and, 113
  gallic acid and, 113
  green tea and, 113
  morin and, 113
  myricetin and, 113
  neurotoxicity, tea extracts and, 110–111
  piceatannol and, 113
  quercetin and, 113
Acetominophen
  elimination, 35
  glucuronidation, 26
  hepatotoxicity, 35
  metabolism, 34
  sulfation, 26, 29
  UGT activity, 27
Aging, 1–5
  biological interaction, 6
  brain, 107–117 (*See also* Brain)
  chronic disease and, 31
  CNS effects, 7–9, 15
  cognitive, 16
  evolutionary theory of, 15
  flavonoid bioavailability and, 19–37
  fundamentals, 3
  genistein levels and, 29
  healthy, 3, 7, 17
  hepatotoxicity and, 34
  liver, 33, 34, 35
  memory and, 9, 16
  neuronal loss and, 8
  phase II metabolism and, 26–28
  physiology of, 6, 15, 17, 24–25, 33
  population, heterogeneity of, 4
  processes, 6
  protein metabolism and, 33
  regenerative responses, 6
  reinterpretation, 3
  retina, 104, 105
  successful, 6, 7, 15
  usual, 6
  xenobiotic metabolism and, 26
Algae, 68, 71

Allergic rhinitis, 185, 186
Allergy
  mediator release, botanicals and, 175–176
  mediators, 176, 185
  prevalence, 173
  prevention, 186
  symptoms, 174, 176
  test botanicals for, 176, 185
  treatment, 184
  wheal sizes, 179
Alzheimer's disease, 7, 8, 107
  amyloid hypothesis of, 115
  diet and, 108, 115
  exercise and, 16
  inflammatory process, 195
  prevention, 114, 116
  resveratrol and, 116
  transgenic mouse model, 116
  treatment, 108
Anisophyllea dichostyla, 56
Anthocyanins, 21, 42, 52–55
Anti-inflammatory botanicals, 77–86, 190–195
Antioxidant(s), 63, 68, 71. *See also* Carotenoid(s);
        Flavonoid(s)
  anticancer activities, 122
  dietary, 151
  NF-κB and, 154
  in pomegranate juice, 151
  in restenosis, 151
  retinitis pigmentosa and, 105
  in vitro, 43, 44
APCI. *See* Atmospheric pressure chemical
        ionization (APCI)
Apigenin, 21
Apo A-I. *See* Apolipoprotein A-I (Apo A-I)
Apo A-IV. *See* Apolipoprotein A-IV (Apo A-IV)
Apolipoprotein A-I (Apo A-I), 156, 158–159, 166
Apolipoprotein A-IV (Apo A-IV), 159–162, 166
APPI. *See* Atmospheric pressure photoionization
        (APPI)
Apples, 47, 48, 55, 56, 58
  isorhamnetin glycosides in extracts of, 76
  juice, pomegranate juice *vs.,* 139, 140
  peel, 74
  quantitation of polyphenols in, 76
Arteriosclerosis, 44, 81
Arthritis, 81, 124, 134
Artichoke leaf extract, 193
Asthma, 81, 185, 186, 187

Milton Keynes UK
Ingram Content Group UK Ltd.
UKHW040100071024
449327UK00019B/704